The Apocrine Glands and the Breast

The Apocrine Glands and the Breast

Marshall B L Craigmyle MB ChB MD

Professor of Anatomy, American University of the Caribbean, Plymouth, Monserrat, British West Indies, formerly Visiting Senior Lecturer, Department of Anatomy, Texas A & M University Medical School, College Station, Texas, U.S.A.

A Wiley Medical Publication

JOHN WILEY & SONS
Chichester · New York · Brisbane · Toronto · Singapore

Library of Congress Cataloging in Publication Data

Craigmyle, M. B. L. (Marshall Buchanan Lang)
The apocrine glands and the breast.

(A Wiley medical publication)
Includes index.
1. Apocrine glands. 2. Mammary glands. I. Title.
II. Series. [DNLM: 1. Breast—anatomy & histology.
2. Breast—growth & development. 3. Sweat Gland Diseases.
4. Sweat Glands—anatomy & histology. 5. Sweat Glands—growth & development. WR 400 C886a[
QM491.C73 1984 612′.664 84–7567
ISBN 0 471 90506 2

British Library Cataloguing in Publication Data

Craigmyle, Marshall B.L.
The apocrine glands and the breast.—
(A Wiley medical publication)
1. Apocrine glands
I. Title
612.4 QP188.A/

ISBN 0 471 90506 2

Typeset by Inforum Ltd., Portsmouth.
Printed by Page Bros. (Norwich) Ltd., Norfolk

Contents

Preface

The apocrine glands have come of age since Hurley & Shelley published their classic book on the glands in health and disease in 1960. My interest in the glands spans the past twelve years, during which time very substantial advances into our knowledge of their form and function have been made. The glands are of general interest to the surgeon because infection of the glands leads to the condition of hidradenitis suppuritiva, which affects primarily the axillary group, but can affect other groups; the glands are also of general interest to the pathologist and the dermatologist. But the studies of the glands have been extremely fragmentary: thus the glands of Moll in the eyelid are seen to be the almost exclusive province of the ophthalmologist and the ceruminous glands of the external acoustic meatus are, by similar general agreement, the concern of the otorhinolaryngologist. The apocrine glands of the external genitalia fall to the urogenital surgeons when diseased, and the obstetrician has the care of the breast in his hands. In this book I have drawn together the information which has been gleaned by these diverse groups, and by others such as the electron microscopists and the biochemists, and blended it to form a cohesive whole account of the glands for what I believe to be the very first time. The book required to be written in the interest of the patient and of the medical profession, and I am happy and privileged to have had the opportunity to do so. I am very convinced that every doctor will find much to interest him within the pages of this little book, and if he does, my efforts will not have been in vain.

M B L Craigmyle
1984

Acknowledgements

The work on which this book is based was carried out in the Department of Anatomy, University College, Cardiff and I am indebted to Professor J D Lever, head of that Department for providing facilities and encouragement during the time I was a member of his staff. I am grateful to Dr William Clee, Dr R Catherine Jones and Miss Alison Rushforth for their help and for permission to reproduce their material. I wish to thank Professor R C Curran, head of the Department of Pathology of the Medical School, University of Birmingham for his constructive criticism. I am indebted to Mrs Pam Whiting for the typing of the manuscript, and to Ms Janet Natowitz for typing the index. Finally, my thanks are due to my wife, Sadie, for her constant encouragement and resultant self-denial during many long winter evenings.

MBLC

PART I

The Apocrine Glands

Chapter 1

Historical Introduction

The discovery of the apocrine glands of the skin is attributed most commonly to Krause (1844). He reported them as occurring in the axilla, the circumanal region and the external acoustic meatus. Accounts of the glands were published almost simultaneously, however, by Rolin (1846) and Horner (1846). By 1853, descriptions of apocrine glands had found their way into the textbooks of histology (von Kölliker) and the first description of apocrine sweat is that by von Kölliker (1853) as a "whitish-yellow tolerably viscid secretion".

In 1867 Moll described the large apocrine glands in the eyelids which still bear his name today. Heynold (1874) gives a further account of the large ceruminous glads of the external acoustic meatus and Krause (1876) of the apocrine glands in several locations. Sattler (1877) mentions, in respect of the glands of Moll, the presence of elastic fibre networks around the secretory segment of the gland, and described contractile cells in the wall of the secretory part. He called these cells fibromuscular. Tartufieri (1880) questioned the ability of these cells to contract, however. Schiefferdecker (1906) reported that the glands of Moll varied widely in form. Contino (1907) confirmed the presence of contractile cells in the wall of the glands of Moll and concluded, from reconstructions of the glands, that the glands were of unbranched tubular form. He also confirmed the presence of elastic fibres in the wall of the secretory segment. Mislawsky (1909) seems to have been the first observer to describe the apocrine glands as exhibiting a secretory cycle, and that cytoplastic detachment is involved. Brinkmann (1908) can lay claim to being the earliest to observe that the apocrine glands do not appear to become functional until after puberty.

It was left, however, to Schiefferdecker (1922) to coin the term apocrine to describe the manner of secretion of the glands as contrasted with the merocrine method of secretion described earlier for the eccrine sweat glands by Ranvier (1887): he described the lining cells of the apocrine glands as forming lingual projections which became pinched off during the secretory process and observed further that for a period thereafter the cells underwent a refractory period during which they could produce only a watery secretion. Schiefferdecker finally described variation in the numbers of apocrine glands with race and sex, facts which were later confirmed by Homma (1926).

Woollard (1930) seems to have been the first to draw the conclusion that apocrine glands are compound tubular as opposed to the simple tubular form of eccrine glands. Horn (1935) and Sperling (1935) concluded independently from wax reconstructions of axillary apocrine glands that they exhibited anastomotic shunts between adjacent coils, and also possessed pouch-like diverticula. Way & Memmesheimer (1938) made out a very good case for designating apocrine glands as accessory sexual glands, a fact with which Higginson & McDonald (1949) strongly agreed. The cytoarchitecture and chemical cytology of apocrine glands were investigated by Bunting (1948) and Bunting *et al.* (1948).

During the last 30 years there have been extensive investigations of the development, form and function of the apocrine glands by Hurley, Shelley and their co-workers (see Hurley & Shelley 1960), by Montagna and his co-workers (see Montagna & Parakkal 1974) and by Hashimoto and his associates, as a result of which much of the mystery surrounding the glands has been dissipated. To this volume of knowledge I wish to add some new facts gleaned from work carried out over the last several years by myself and some of my students (Clee 1975; Jones 1977; Rushforth 1982).

REFERENCES

Brinkmann A (1908) Die Rückendrüsen von Dicotyles. *Z. Anat Entwicklung*, **36**, 281–307

Bunting H (1948) Cytochemical properties of apocrine sweat glands normally present in the human mammary gland. *Anat Rec*, **101**, 5–12

Bunting, H, Wislocki G B & Dempsey E W (1948) The chemical histology of human eccrine and apocrine sweat glands. *Anat Rec*, **100**, 61–78

Carlini V (1907) *Il Tessuto Elastico.* In: Rapporto con le Ghiandolle di Moll. *Ann Ottal*, **36**, 231–234

Clee W B (1975) *A Study of the Modified or Apocrine Sweat Glands of Human Skin.* BSc Thesis, University of Wales

Contino A (1907) *Graefes Arch Clin Exp Ophthalmol*, **66**, 505

Heynold H (1874) *Virchows Arch (Pathol Anat)*, **61** 77 (cited by Hurley & Shelley 1960)

Higginson J F & McDonald J R (1949) Apocrine tissue, chronic cystic mastitis and sweat gland carcinoma of the breast. *Surg Gynecol Obstet*, **88**, 1–10

Homma H (1926) On apocrine glands in white and negro women. *Bull Johns Hopkins Hosp*, **38**, 365–371

Horn G (1935) Formentwicklung und Gestalt der Schweissdrüsen Fussole des Menschen *Z Mikrosk Anat Forsch*, **38**, 318–329

Horner W E (1846) On the odiferous glands of the negro. *Am J Med Sci*, **21**, 13–16

Hurley H J & Shelley W B (1960) *The Human Apocrine Sweat Gland in Health and Disease*. Springfield, Ill: Charles C Thomas

Jones R C (1977) *A Study of the Glands of Moll in the Fetus and Adult*. BSc Thesis, University of Wales

Kölliker A von (1853) In: *Manual of Human Histology*, eds G Busk & T Hurley. London: Sydenham Society

Krause C (1844) Die Haut. In: *Wagner's Handbook of Physiology*, **2**, 108 (cited by Hurley & Shelley 1960)

Krause W (1876) *Handbuch der Menschlichen Anatomie*. Berlin: Erster Bond (cited by Woolard 1930)

Mislawsky A N (1909) Zur Lehre von der sogennanten blasenförmigen Sekretion. *Arch Mikrosk Anat*, **73**, 681–689

Moll J A (1867) Bemerkungen über den Bander Augenlider des Menschen. *Arch Ophthalmol*, **3**, 258–268

Montagna W & Parakkal P F (1974) *The Structure and Function of Skin*. New York: Academic Press

Ranvier (1877) cited by Kuno Y (1956) *Human Perspiration*. Springfield, Ill: Charles C Thomas

Rolin C (1846) Sudoriparous glands of the axilla. *Am J Med Sci*, **11**, 436

Rushforth A (1982) *On the Sweat Glands of the Face and of the Areola*. BSc Thesis, University of Wales

Sattler H (1877) Beitrag zür Kenntnis der modificirten Mollschen Schweissdrüsen des Lidrandes. *Arch Mikrosk Anat*, **13**, 783–795

Schiefferdecker P (1906) Die drüsen des menschlichen Augenlides. *Dtsch Med Wochenschr Berlin*, **32**, 1886–1887

Schiefferdecker P (1922) Die Hautdrüsen des menschen. *Zoologica*, **27**, 1–154

Sperling G (1925) Die Form der apocrinen Hautdrüsen des menschen. *Z Mikrosk Anat Forsch*, **38**, 241–252

Tartufieri A (1880) Le ghiandole di Moll studiate velle palpebre dell ums e degli altri mammiferi e comparate alle tubulare cutanee. *Arch Sci Med (Torino)*, **4**

Way S C & Memmesheimer A (1938) The sudoriparous glands. II The apocrine glands. *Arch Dermatol Syphilol*, **38**, 373–382

Woollard H (1930) The cutaneous glands of man. *J Anat*, **64**, 415–421

Chapter 2

The Development of the Apocrine Glands

There have been considerable numbers of studies of the development of the apocrine glands in several locations and this account is based on the following: Sattler 1877; Contino 1907; Carossini 1912; Steiner 1926; Borsetto 1951; Pinkus 1958; Montagna 1959; Nishio 1964; Hashimoto 1970; Jones 1977.

Apocrine glands develop from ectodermal downgrowths known as apo-pilo-sebaceous units, in distinct contrast to eccrine glands which arise from the surface ectoderm at large. The apo-pilo-sebaceous units have, by the fifth month of intra-uterine life, differentiated sufficiently as to be recognisable as primitive hair follicles which run to the skin surface at an angle. Each of these hair follicles will develop two bulges on that side of the follicle which forms an obtuse angle with the surface. The deeper of these bulges marks the site of attachment of the developing arrector pili muscle, and the more superficial bulge is the primordium of the sebaceous glands of that follicle. Where a primitive hair follicle is to form an apocrine gland, a third bulge will be seen superficial to the other two and at the junction of the hair follicle and the surface epidermis. (According to Hurley & Shelley, 1960, such a bulge forms on every hair follicle in all regions, but regresses in those areas where apocrine glands do not form.) At the time when the apocrine bud is starting to make its appearance, the eccrine glands are already in a fairly advanced state of development. According to Homma (1926) eccrine glands may subsequently become translocated from the surface to the wall of the hair follicle whereas the reverse never occurs – ie. apocrine glands never open to the skin surface but eccrine glands do sometimes open into hair follicles.

The apocrine bud is a solid mass of epithelial cells and by the sixth fetal month it has reached the deep part of the dermis and has started to coil. At about the same time the central cells in the superficial part of the bud start to degenerate so as to form a lumen: this process extends peripherally and by the seventh or eighth month, canalisation is complete throughout the length of the bud. At this stage the apocrine gland buds are larger in diameter than their eccrine counterparts and the deep extremity is expanded so that the profile, in cross section, is that of an alveolus lined by stratified cuboidal epithelium. At birth the apocrine glands, however, are smaller than the eccrine glands (Montagna 1959) but at all times they have a much larger lumen than eccrine glands, whose profile on section is that of an acinus.

The apocrine glands remain smaller than the eccrine glands until about the fourth year of life when they start to enlarge, the process starting earlier in girls than in boys. By the age of seven or eight, the gland has acquired all the criteria diagnostic of ability to secrete (Montes *et al.* 1960): thus, the lining cells may now be columnar, with microvilli and psuedopodia, and a clear band of apical cytoplasm. Further, cytoplasmic basophilia, supranuclear PAS-positive granules and PAS positivity in the brush border are all present. Around this time, too, the myoepithelium becomes recognisable as such in that myofibrils now make their appearance in the basal cells. The ceruminous glands of the external acoustic meatus are functional at birth according to Hurley & Shelley (1960) but Perry (1957) says, on the other hand, that they do not become functional until puberty.

REFERENCES

Borsetto P S (1951) Observazione sullo sviluppo delle ghiandole sudoripare nelle diverse regione della cute umana. *Arch Ital Anat Embriol*, **56**, 332–348

Carossini G (1912) Lo sviluppo delle ghiandole sudoripara particolamente ne' suoi rapporti collo sviluppo dell' apparato pilifer, nelle diverse regioni della pelle dell' uoma. *Arch Ital Anat Embriol*, **11**, 545–603

Contino A (1907) *Graefes Arch Clin Exp Ophthalmol*, **66**, 505

Hashimoto K (1970) The ultrastructure of the skin of human embryos. VII Formation of the apocrine gland. *Acta Derm Venereol (Stockh)*, **50**, 241–251

Homma H (1926) On apocrine glands in white and negro women. *Bull Johns Hopk Hosp*, **38**, 365–371

Hurley H J & Shelley W B (1960) *The Human Apocrine Sweat Gland in Health and Disease*. Springfield, Ill: Charles C Thomas

Jones R C (1977) *A Study of the Glands of Moll in the Fetus and Adult*. BSc Thesis, University of Wales

Montagna W (1959) Histology and cytochemistry of human skin. XIX The development and fate of the axilliary organ. *J Invest Dermatol*, **33**, 151–156

Montes L F, Baker B L & Curtis A C (1960) The cytology of the large axilliary sweat glands in man. *J Invest Dermatol*, **35**, 273–291

Nishio T (1964) Embryological studies on the apocrine sweat glands in the whole body of Japanese. *J Yonago Med Assoc*, **15**, 185–208

Perry E T (1957) *The Human Ear Canal*. Springfield, Ill: Charles C Thomas
Pinkus H (1958) Embryology of hair. In: *Biology of Hair Growth*, eds W Montagna & R A Ellis. New York: Academic Press
Sattler H (1877) Beitrag zür Kenntnis der modificirten Mollschen Schweissdrüsen des Lidrandes. *Arch Mikrosk Anat*, **13**, 783–795
Steiner K (1926) Über die Entwicklung der grossen Schweissdrüsen beim menschen. *Z Anat Entwicklung*, **78**, 83–97

Chapter 3

The Anatomy of the Apocrine Glands

Definition

Apocrine glands may be defined as being those 'sweat' glands (Fig 1; Table 1) in which:

1. the secretory tubule exhibits branching (as compared with the eccrine sweat gland in which the tubule does not branch);
2. the secretory tubule, as seen in cross-section is of alveolar form (as

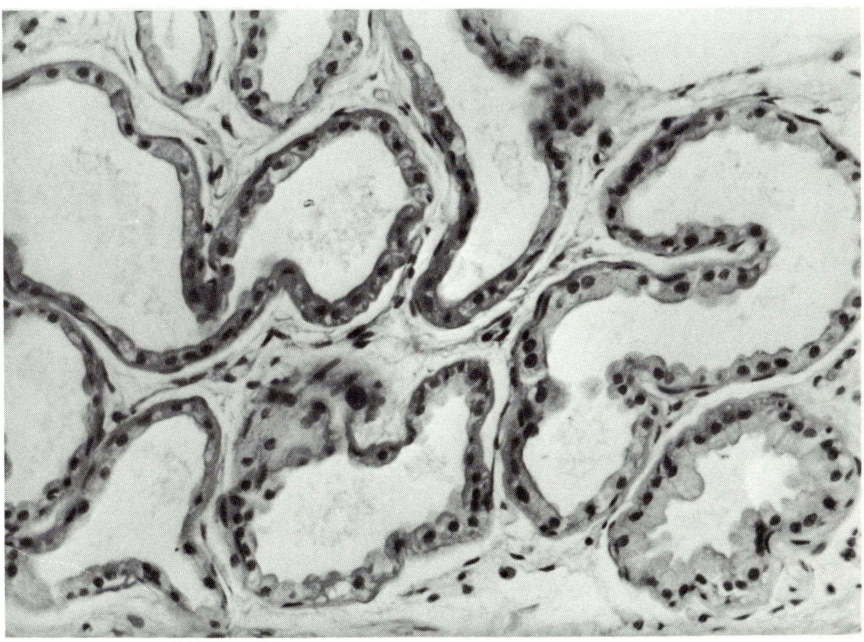

Fig 1 *Axillary apocrine gland.* The gland profiles are lined by a simple epithelium which may be squamous or cuboidal or columnar. Only one type of secretory cell is present. Myoepithelial cells are to be seen (arrows). The lumen is wide. The tubules branch and have diverticula. H & E × 700.

Table 1 Comparison of Apocrine and Eccrine Glands

	Apocrine	Eccrine
Gland type	Branched	Unbranched
Cross-sectional appearance of secretory portion	Alveolar-like	Acinar-like
Type of lining epithelium of secretory portion	Simple	Pseudostratified
Number of cell types in secretory portion	One	Two (clear and dark)
Myoepithelium	Present	Present
Manner of secretion	Merocrine Apocrine Holocrine	Merocrine
Type of duct epithelium	Stratified cuboidal	Stratified cuboidal
Passage of duct through epidermis	Straight	Coiled
Location of duct opening	Wall of hair follicle	Skin surface
Direction of duct in dermis	At an angle to surface	Perpendicular to surface
Nature of duct in dermis	Often coiled	Straight

distinct from the acinar form of a cross-section of the tubule of eccrine glands);

3. the lining epithelium of the secretory segment is simple squamous, simple cuboidal or simple columnar (as opposed to the pseudo-stratified columnar epithelial lining of eccrine glands); and
4. only one cell type is to be found in the secretory segment (as contrasted with the two cell types, clear and dark, found in eccrine sweat glands); myoepithelial cells found in both gland types.

Distribution

Apocrine glands are of widespread occurrence. Their presence is widely documented in some regions – suprapubic region, circumanal region, axilla and umbilical region. In other areas they have been reported as being present by some investigators and as absent by others. They have at one time or another been described as being present in skin from the following areas:

1 Axilla
2 Umbilical region
3 Suprapubic region
4 Circumanal region
5 Hairy part of chest (Szodoray 1948)
6 Areola (Bunting 1948)
7 Hypogastric region (Vohwinkel 1931)
8 Inguinal region (Hurley & Shelley 1960)
9 Prepuce (Montagna 1962)
10 Scrotum (Sobotta/Hammersen 1980)
11 Labium majus (Hewer/Foster 1969)
12 Labium minus (Montagna 1962)
13 Scalp (Pinkus 1958)
14 Eyebrow (Hashimoto 1970)
15 Malar region (Hurley & Shelley 1960)
16 Forehead (Vohwinkel 1931)
17 Bearded portion of face (Pinkus 1958)
18 Nasal vestibule (Alverdes 1932)
19 Scalp (Szodoray 1948)
To these must be added:
20 The glands of Moll in the eyelids
21 The ceruminous glands of the cartilaginous part of the external acoustic meatus
22 The breast (Higginson & McDonald 1949).

Indeed, Homma (1926) goes so far as to state that they may be found wherever hairy skin occurs and that the only sites where they are not encountered are the palms of the hands and soles of the feet but I am not aware of any reference to their presence elsewhere in the limbs. Certainly, the embryologists are of the opinion that apocrine buds may form in all hair follicles and that in the face and scalp buds form on the majority. It does not seem reasonable to describe as ectopic (Szordoray 1948) those apocrine glands located in skin other than that of the axilla, the inguinal region, the perianal area, the areola, the umbilicus, the eyelid, the ear and the hairy part of the chest since there are as many ectopic regions as non-ectopic ones under this classification: there is disagreement further, between later investigators, as to which groups are ectopic and which are not.

GROSS STRUCTURE

The apocrine gland is about 10 times larger than the eccrine (Horner 1846) and is of yellow or yellow-brown colour. Apocrine glands are of compound tubular form (Woollard 1930; Sperling 1935; Horn 1935; Clee 1975; Jones 1977) and distinct from eccrine glands which are, by

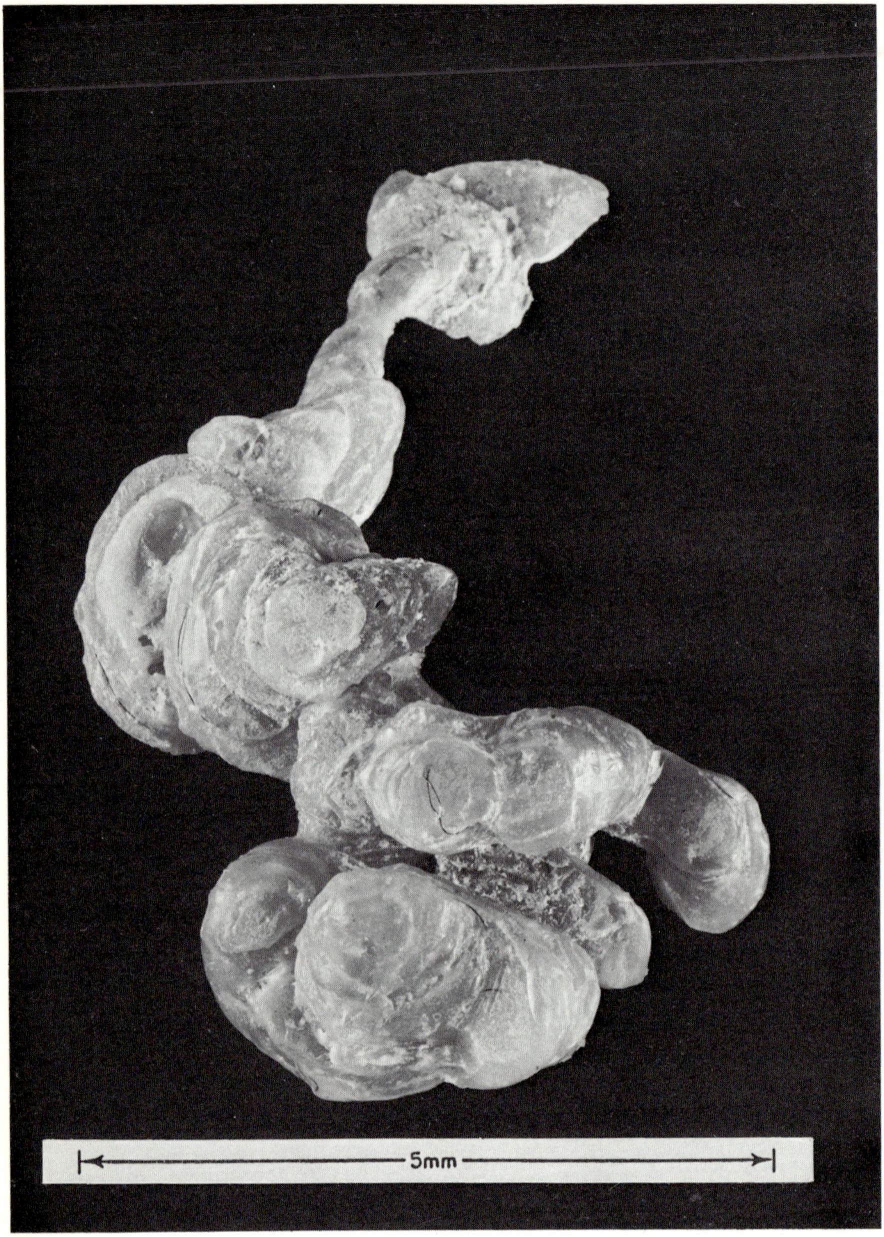

Fig 2 *Gland of Moll.* The gland branches and exhibits diverticula. Reconstruction by Dr R Catherine Jones.

universal acclaim, of simple tubular form. The apocrine glands consist of a deep, coiled portion and a straight portion running to the skin surface: the coiled portion, in the largest glands of the axilla, may be seen readily by the naked eye since it attains a diameter of 1–2 mm. The coiled portion is 50 mm long and 3–5 mm wide (Woollard 1930). The coiled portion is located deep in the dermis, or in the subcutis, or at the junction of the two: it may be as much as 5 mm from the skin surface (Montagna & Parakkal 1974). The bulk of the coil comprises the secretory segment of the gland, and continuity with the duct portion may occur within, or at the edge of, the coiled portion. The transition from secretory portion to duct portion is abrupt, and is readily recognised because of the greater diameter of the secretory portion compared with that of the duct.

The secretory portions of axillary apocrine glands were reconstructed by Sperling (1935) and Horn (1935) and shown to possess diverticuli, and shunts between adjacent coils. We can confirm this for the axillary glands and have found shunts and diverticuli in the apocrine glands from the suprapubic and circumanal regions (Clee 1975), in the glands of Moll (Jones 1977) (Fig 2) and in the glands of the areola (Rushforth 1982) (Fig 3). The axillary glands are unquestionably the most complex: the suprapubic and circumanal glands are of an intermediate degree of complexity and the glands of Moll are the least complex: indeed, the majority of the glands in the last group do not exhibit shunts or diverticuli. We can also confirm Contino's observation (1907) that the glands of Moll may exhibit two secretory coils: they are, however, much smaller than the axillary glands and their degree of coiling is also much less.

Diverticuli arise most commonly from the deepest parts of the glands. The various forms of diverticuli seen by us in axillary glands are illustrated in Fig 4.

Ducts of apocrine glands differ from eccrine ducts in the following respects:

(i) Apocrine ducts open almost invariably into a hair follicle whereas eccrine ducts open onto the skin surface. Apocrine glands open very occasionally however onto the skin surface (eg. in the areola and in the labium minus) and the duct orifice is then surrounded by sebaceous glands.

(ii) Apocrine ducts run towards the surface at an angle, and parallel to the hair follicles of the region. Eccrine ducts are usually perpendicular to the skin surface.

(iii) The apocrine duct is straight and wide (infundibulum) where it penetrates the epidermis of the side wall of a hair follicle. Eccrine ducts are narrow and highly-coiled as they pass through the epidermis of the skin surface.

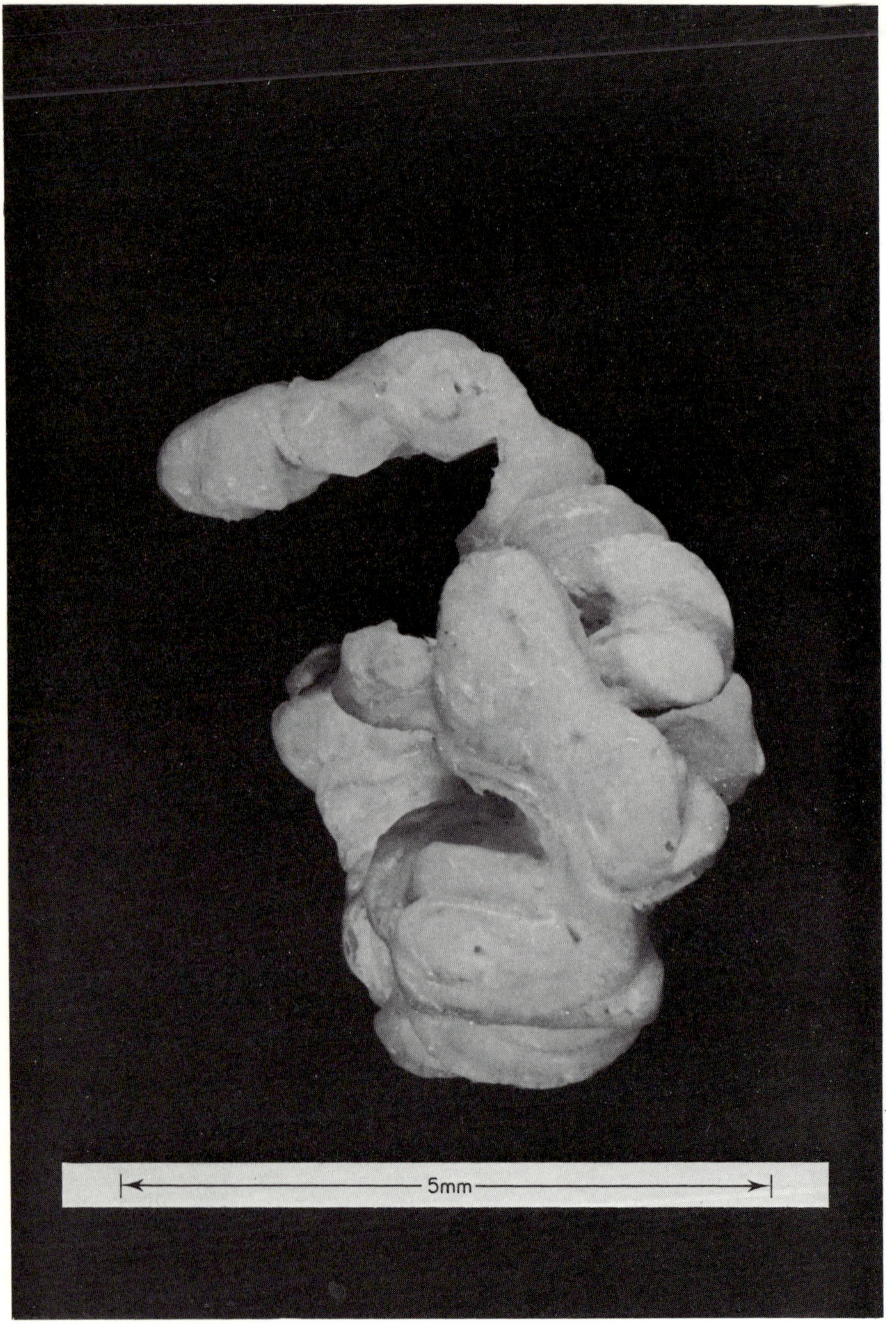

Fig 3 *Areolar apocrine gland*. The gland exhibits branching and possesses diverticula. Reconstruction by Miss A Rushforth

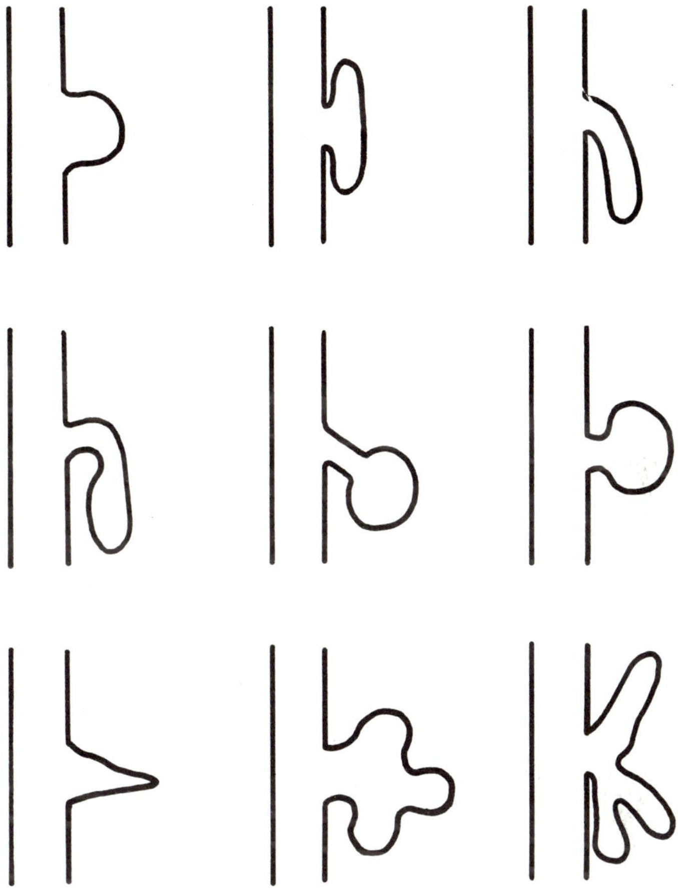

Fig 4 *Types of diverticula seen in axillary apocrine glands*. Drawing by Dr William Clee

(iv) Apocrine ducts may have a loop or even a coil: eccrine ducts never do.

Hair follicles with one, two or perhaps three apocrine glands opening into them can be seen in the axilla, the suprapubic area and the circumanal region: the same is true of eyelash follicles and numbers of glands of Moll. The majority of hair follicles in all these regions will, however, have no associated apocrine gland.

The ratio of eccrine glands to apocrine glands in a given location is difficult to estimate because of the enormous degree of individual variation in the presence and the numbers of apocrine glands in most regions. In the axilla, however, where it would appear that apocrine glands are universally present, it is claimed on one hand (Hurley & Shelley 1960) that there are four or five times as many eccrine as apocrine glands and on the other (Montagna & Parakkal 1974) that the two types are found in equal numbers.

HISTOLOGICAL STRUCTURE

The Secretory Segment

The secretory segment of apocrine glands is lined by a simple epithelium in which only one type of cell is to be found. The lining cells may be squamous (Fig 5), cuboidal (Fig 6) or columnar (Fig 7). Spindle-shaped myoepithelial cells (Fig 8) lie between the lining cells and the conspicuous basement membrane. The diameter of the lumen ranges from 50 to 400 microns and of the secretory profile from 50 to 450 microns (Fig 9).

In studies of apocrine glands from the axilla, the suprapubic region and the circumanal region (Clee 1975) and the glands of Moll (Jones 1977) we have found that the height of the epithelium in any one apocrine gland is usually a constant. Thus, in 168 serially-sectioned apocrine glands from the above four regions, 122 (73%) have a lining which is constant for the length of the gland: of these 41 (34%) had a squamous linind, 37 (30%) had a cuboidal lining and 44 (36%) had a columnar lining. Of the 46 serially-sectioned apocrine glands in which the epithelial height was not constant, 13 had an epithelium which was either squamous or cuboidal and 17 were lined by an epithelium which varied from cuboidal to columnar. In only 16 (11%) of the serially-sectioned apocrine glands did the lining epithelium exhibit all three heights. Adjacent glands may have a different lining, and glands of all four lining types (ie. squamous, cuboidal, columnar or mixed) have been seen in the eyelid, axilla, suprapubic region and circumanal region. In mixed glands, there is no consistent arrangement of the various epithelial heights: thus the highest epithelium can be seen, for example, in the proximal, the distal or the intermediate sector of the secretory tubule.

The epithelium lining a diverticulum (Fig 10) is usually of the same height as, but may be of a different height from, the epithelium lining the secretory segment from which the diverticulum has arisen. We have seen squamous epithelium in diverticula originating from a secretory segment lined by columnar epithelium, and vice-versa. The diverticuli have a luminal diameter which, in general, is about half that of the secretory coil from which they arise. We have seen, in one axillary gland, a diverticulum arising from an apocrine duct.

The lining cells possess a brush border (Minimatani 1941). Apical

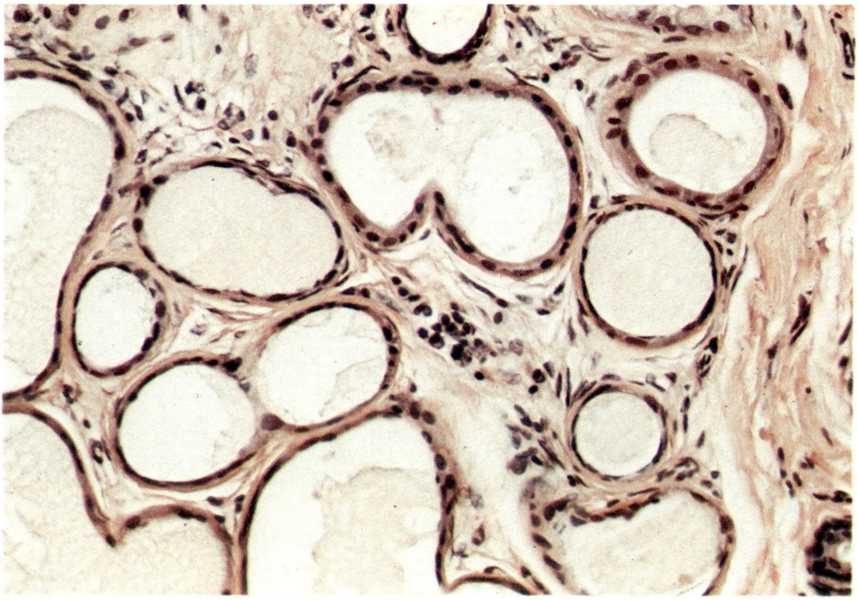

Fig 5 *Axillary apocrine gland.* The gland profiles are lined for the most part by simple squamous epithelium. H & E × 800

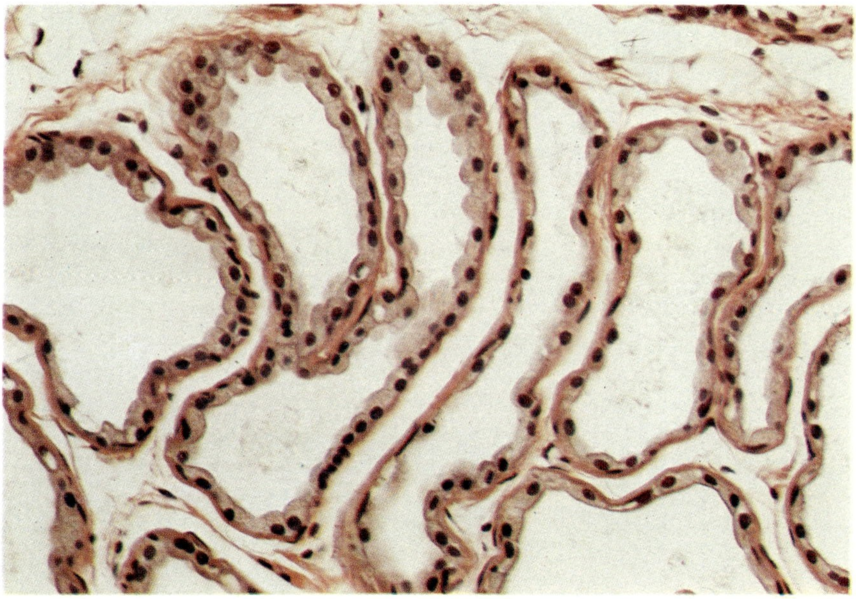

Fig 6 *Axillary apocrine gland.* The predominant type of lining is simple cuboidal. H & E × 800

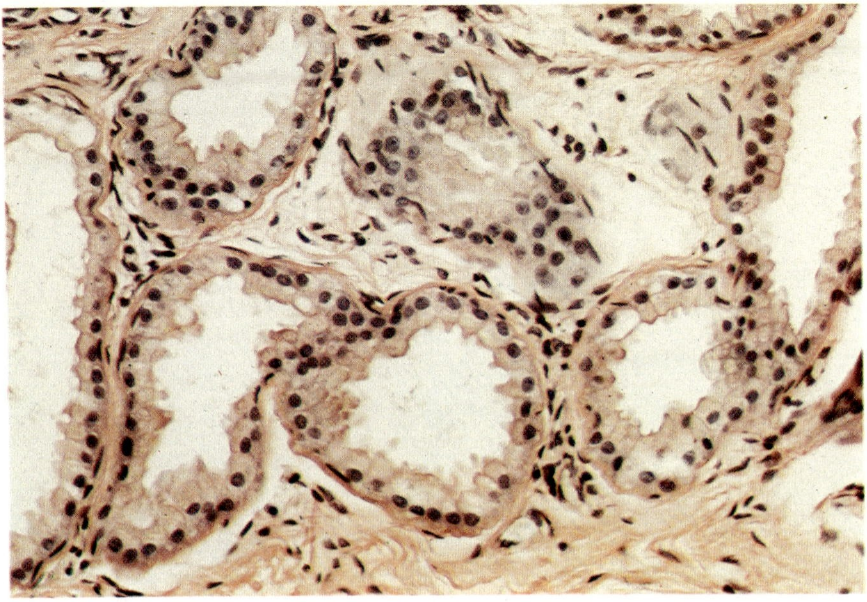

Fig 7 *Axillary apocrine gland.* The gland is lined by a simple columnar epithelium: the lining cells lack apical pseudopodia. H & E × 800

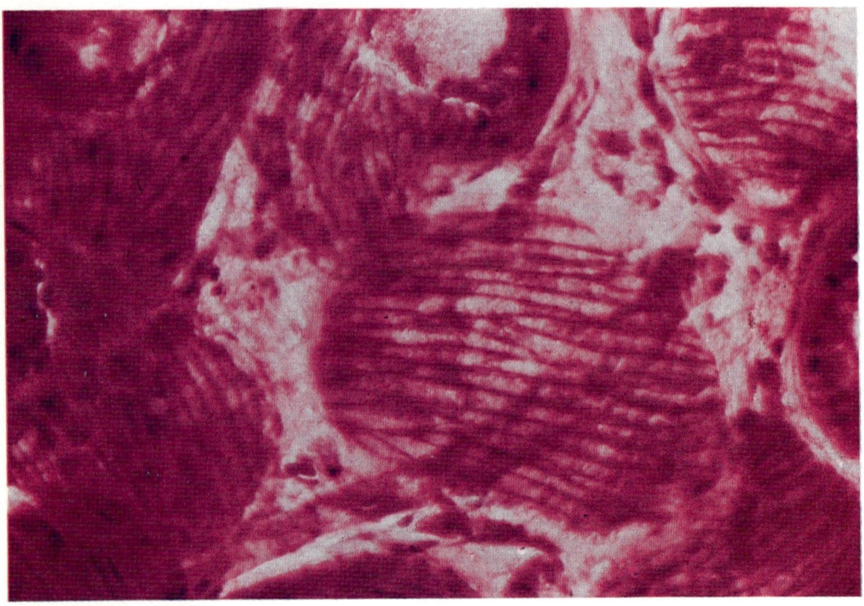

Fig 8 *Axillary apocrine gland.* The myoepithelial cells surrounding the secretory tubule are seen to be narrow and elongated. H & E × 800

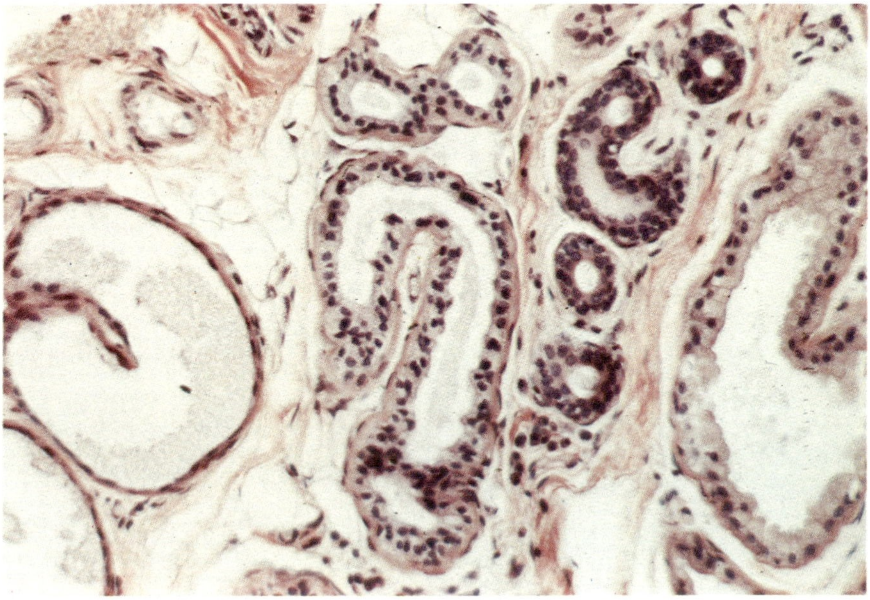

Fig 9 *Axillary apocrine glands*. The luminal diameter is widest in glands in which the lining epithelium is squamous and narrowest in glands with a columnar lining. Duct profiles lined by stratified cuboidal epithelium can also be seen. H & E × 500

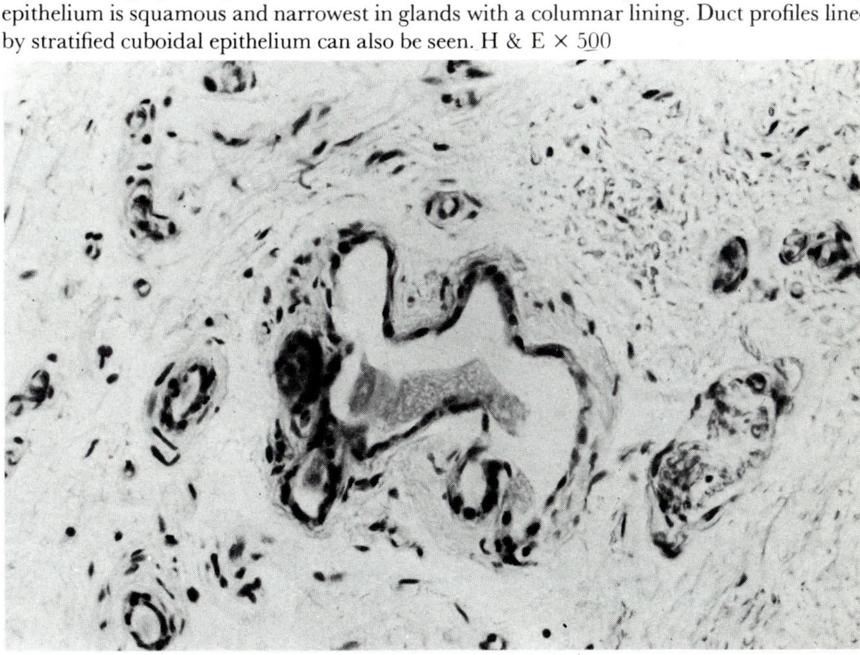

Fig 10 *Apocrine gland in nasal vestibule*. The secretory portion of the gland is lined by simple squamous epithelium and exhibits several diverticula. H & E × 400

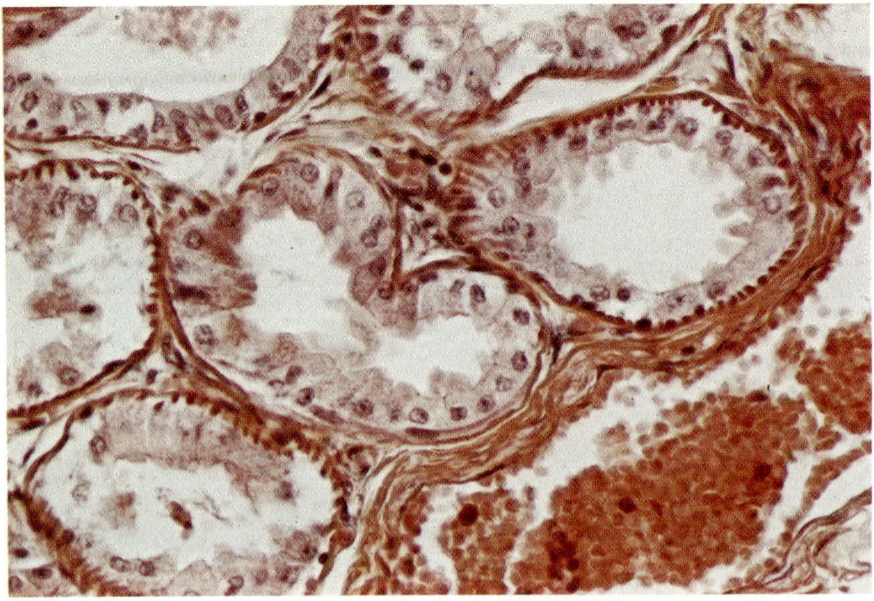

Fig 11 *Axillary apocrine gland.* The lining of the secretory part is simple columnar and the majority of the columnar cells possess apical pseudopodia. H & E × 850

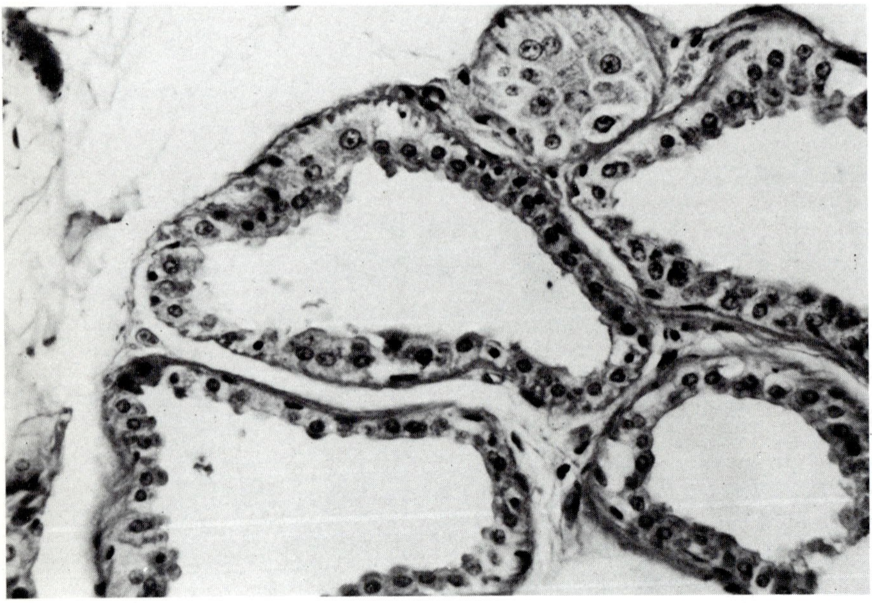

Fig 12 *Axillary apocrine gland.* The secretory profiles are lined by a simple columnar epithelium lacking apical pseudopodia. H & E × 850

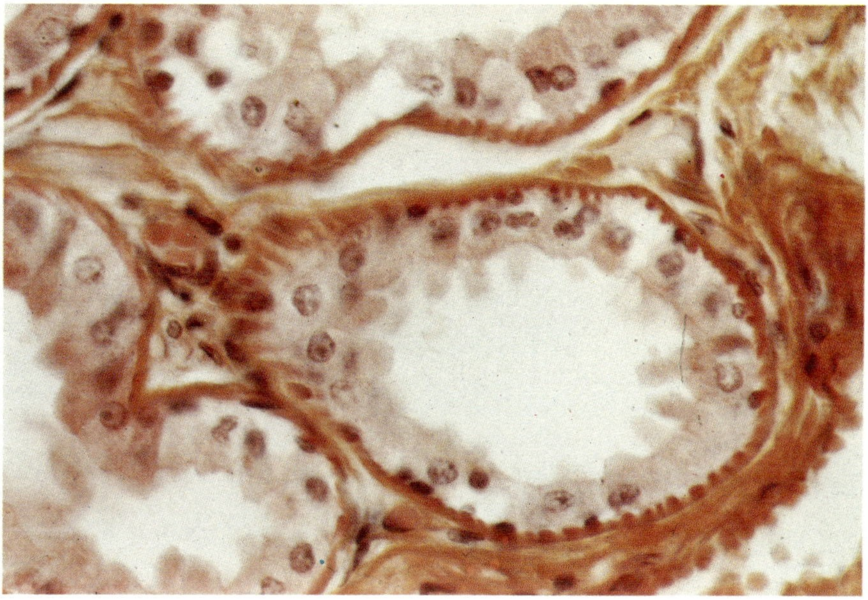

Fig 13 *Axillary apocrine gland.* The apical cytoplasm is amorphous. H & E × 1250

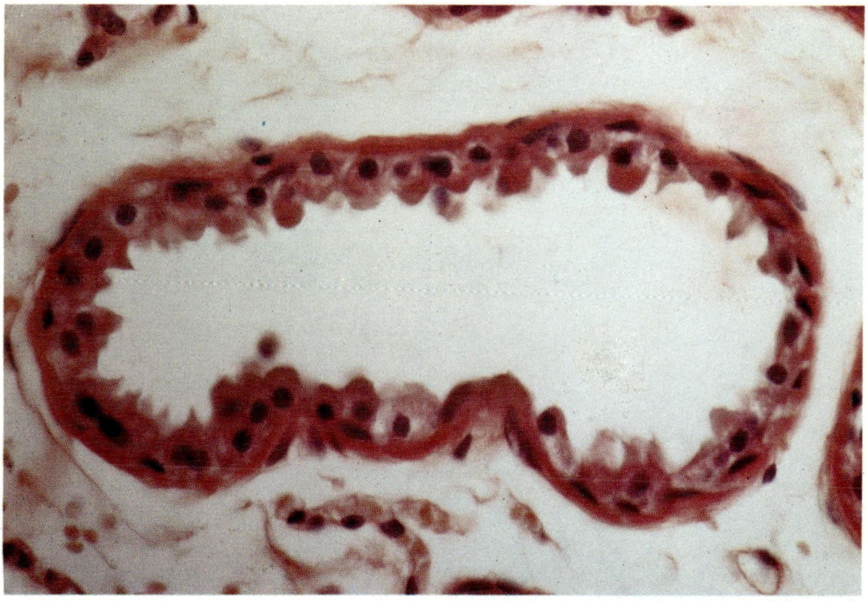

Fig 14 *Axillary apocrine gland.* The pseudopodia contain amorphous cytoplasm. H & E × 1250

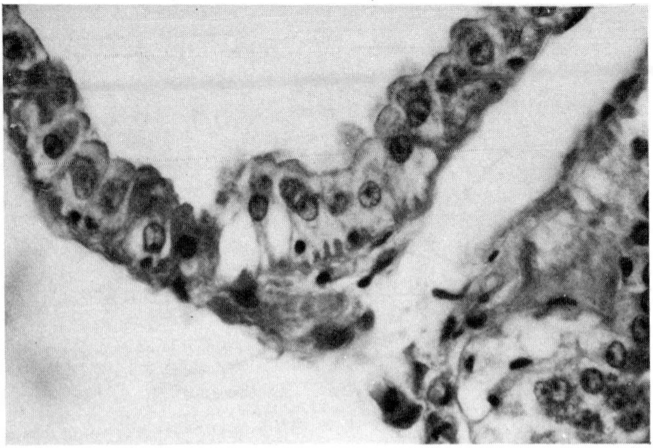

Fig 15 *Axillary apocrine gland*. The brush border exhibits P A S – positivity. P A S × 900

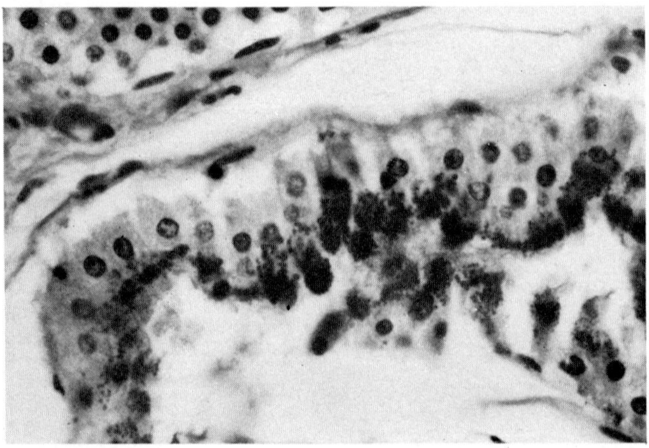

Fig 16 *Axillary apocrine gland*. Supranuclear cytoplasmic granules may be seen, as here, but they never extend into the apical band of amorphous cytoplasm. H & E × 900

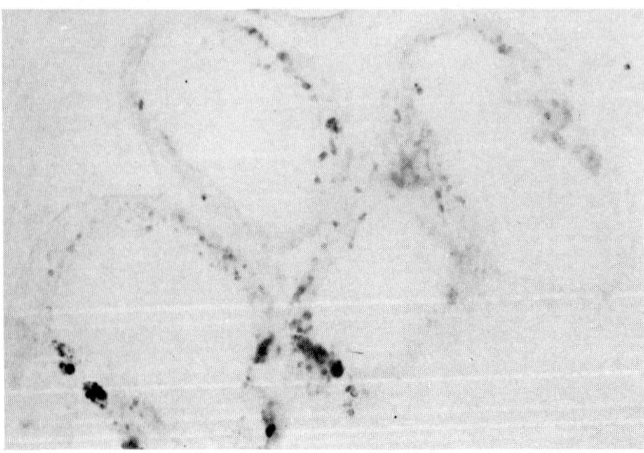

Fig 17 *Axillary apocrine gland*. Unstained preparation. Pigmented secretory granules can be seen in the apical cytoplasm. H & E × 600

Fig 18 *Axillary apocrine gland*. The luminal secretion is finely granular. H & E × 300

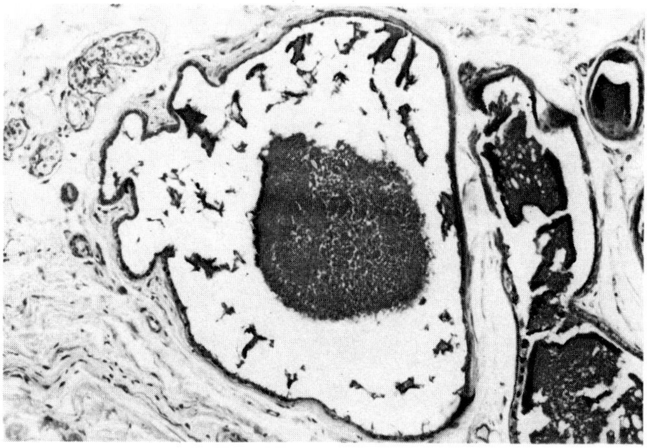

Fig 19 *Axillary apocrine gland*. The luminal secretion is intensely P A S – positive. P A S × 300

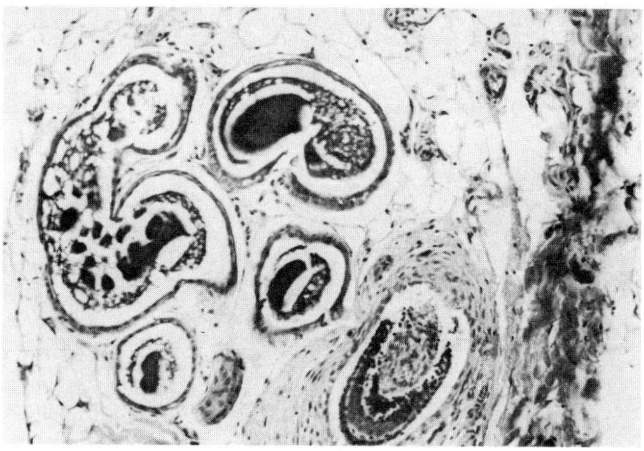

Fig 20 *Axillary apocrine gland*. The myoepithelial cells surround the secretory segment on the left. H & E × 600

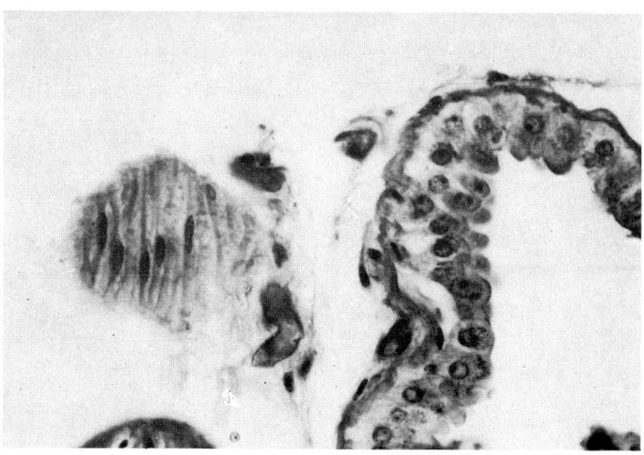

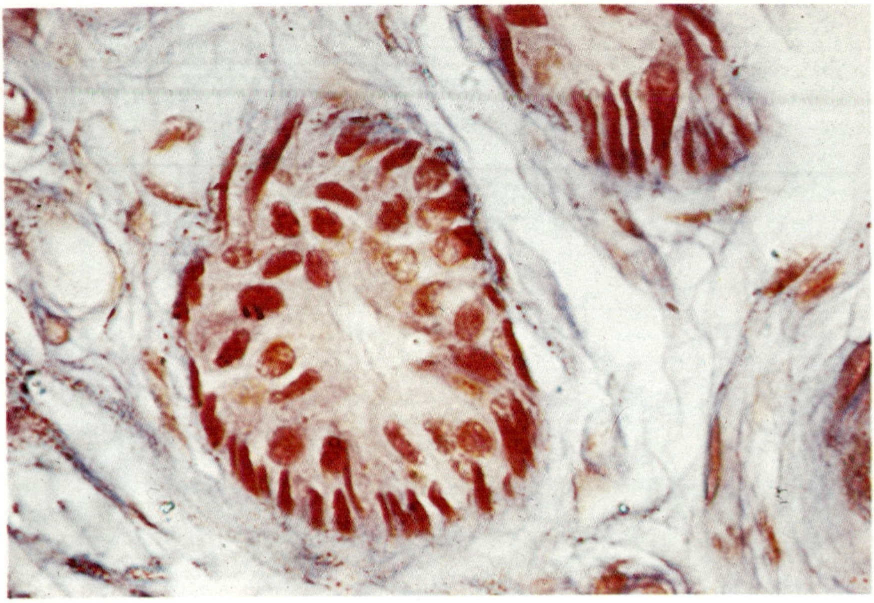

Fig 21 *Axillary apocrine gland*. The basement membrane shows deep infoldings which appear as dark slashes between the bases of the secretory cells. H & E × 1250

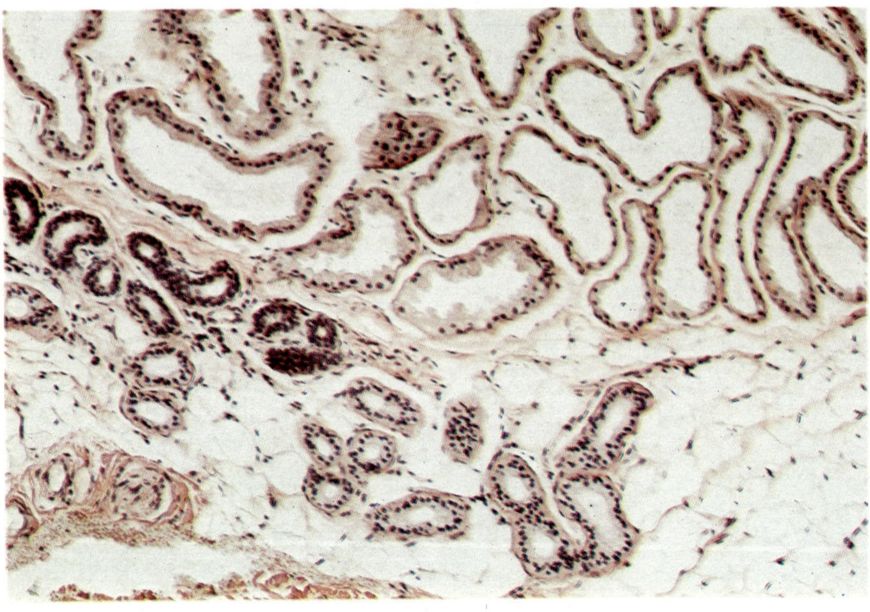

Fig 22 *Axillary apocrine gland (same subject as in Fig 9)*. The duct (centre left) is lined by stratified cuboidal epithelium. H & E × 400

pseudopodia can be seen only atop columnar cells, (Fig 11) but many columnar cells lack this feature (Fig 12). When a pseudopodium is present, the brush border is usually absent, or seen at most at the base of the pseudopodium. In general, columnar-cell-lined profiles either will have pseudopodia all around their circumference, or have no pseudopodia at all.

Cytological Features of the Secretory Segment

The lining cells of the secretory segment have a single deeply-staining nucleus which, in cuboidal or columnar cells, is of spherical outline and located at the base of the cell. In squamous cells the nucleus is ovoid with its long axis parallel to the basement membrane. Binucleate cells are seen occasionally. There are one or two distinct nucleoli.

The cytoplasm of the apocrine gland cell is of a pale pink colour in haematoxylin and eosin-stained preparations, but patches of basophilia are to be seen near the base of the cell. When this basophilia is present in any degree, the nucleus usually lies further from the base of the cell than is usual: further, pronounced basophilia is found in those cells which have few secretory granules (Montes *et al.* 1960). Most columnar cells possess an apical band of cytoplasm which is unstained and devoid of all cell inclusions (Fig 13). This region frequently stains with osmic acid and possesses a "canalicular system" (Montes *et al.* 1960). The pseudopodia, when present, are full of this organelle-deficient cytoplasm (Fig 14). A brush border is present on every cell (Minimatani 1941). On columnar cells with pseudopodia, the brush border is more pronounced on the sides of the pseudopodium than on its summit. The brush border stains intensely PAS-positive (Fig 15) in sharp contrast to the apical cytoplasm (Montes *et al.* 1960). Vesicles can be seen in relation to both the apex and base of the brush border. The basal and lateral plasma membranes of the cells are highly infolded and terminal bars are to be seen near the luminal aspect of the latter. The prominent Golgi apparatus occupies a supranuclear position. It is spherical in columnar cells and flat in squamous cells.

Mitochondria of elongated form occupy the recesses of the unfolded basal plasma membrane: elsewhere the mitochondria are spherical or ovoid and in the supranuclear cytoplasm they may be very large. They are never to be seen in the Golgi region or in the apical cytoplasmic band but may be found in all other parts of the cell.

Eosinophilic secretory granules are present in many of the lining cells (Fig 16). They lie mostly in a supranuclear position although they too are never seen in the Golgi zone or in the apical cytoplasmic band: when present in large numbers, they can be seen flanking the nucleus (Montes *et al.* 1960). Some of the granules are pigmented, others are not (Fig 17); all are PAS-positive (Montagna *et al.* 1953). The granules vary greatly in size, shape, staining intensity and numbers, with the result that reports as to their origin and fate are highly conflicting. We are of the opinion that the relationship of PAS-positive granules to height of cell is difficult to summarise if for no reason other than that such granules can be present in some cells and absent in others within the same profile. We think, however, that in general:

1. squamous cells lack PAS-positive granules;
2. cuboidal cells may have either a sparse complement of PAS-positive granules or a PAS-positive brush border; and
3. columnar cells may have either abundant PAS-positive granules or a PAS-positive brush border.

Apical pseudopodia may be seen in columnar cells possessing granules and in columnar cells which do not: granules will tend to be concentrated in the supranuclear region whether the cell possesses a pseudopodium or not.

The luminal secretion, when present, is in our opinion neither heterogeneous as some have claimed nor homogeneous as has been stated by others, but finely granular (Fig 18). It is intensely PAS-positive (Fig 19), and is constantly present in profiles lined by squamous epithelium – in such profiles the luminal diameter is often greatly in excess ($<600\boldsymbol{m}$) of that seen in profiles lined by columnar or cuboidal cells. This has led many investigators to conclude that duct occlusion is the reason for such accumulations: we are of the opinion that it is seen with such a degree of regularity as to constitute a normal feature.

As to the other cytological and histochemical features of the secretory cells of apocrine glands, a similar diversity of opinion exists. Glycogen is reportedly present in ceruminous (Montagna 1948) and inguinal glands (Hurley & Shelley 1960) but not in glands from other regions (Montagna *et al.* 1951, 1953). Homma (1926) and Manca (1934) reported that iron is present in most apocrine glands whereas Kligman & Shehadeh (1964) say it is sparse in the glands of the mons pubis: Higginson & McDonald (1949) and Montagna & Parakkal (1974) are in agreement that some specimens abound in it whilst others have little or none and that different coils of the same gland contain differing amounts: when iron is present it occurs only in the "pigmented" cells, whatever their height.

Lipids, as detected by the Sudan dyes, are present in the small pigmented granules especially, in the large pigmented granules to some extent but not at all in the non-pigmented granules (Montagna & Parakkal 1974).

Apocrine gland cells show, in addition, the following enzymes:

1 Moderate succinic dehydogenase activity (Montagna & Formisano (1955)
2 Abundant cytochrome oxidase activity (Montagna & Parakkal 1974)
3 Plentiful monoamine oxidase (Yasuda & Montagna 1960)
4 Abundant non-specific esterase (Montagna & Ellis 1958, 1959)
5 ATP-ase activity (Montagna & Parakkal 1974)
6 Alkaline phosphatase activity in the apical border of the tall epithelial cells (Montagna & Parakkal 1974)
7 Acid phosphatase activity in the apical cytoplasm (Montagna & Parakkal 1974)
8 Alpha glucan phosphorylase activity (Sasai 1969)
9 Strong adenosine triphosphatase activity in the basal region (Biempica & Montes 1965).

The Myoepithelium

Spindle-shaped myoepithelial cells are interposed between the bases of the secretory cells and the basement membrane (Fig 20). The similarity of myoepithelium to, and its ability to contract as does, smooth muscle are now accepted so universally that I shall not repeat the arguments here. The myoepithelial cells are disposed with their long axis running lengthwise with respect to the tubule (Bunting *et al.* 1948). The intervals between the myoepithelial cells are occupied by infoldings of the plasma membrane of the basal region of the secretory cells. Hurley & Shelley (1954, 1960) report that peristaltic contractile waves have been seen to pass along the tubule.

The myoepithelial cell cytoplasm stains well with acid dyes: elongated cytoplasmic filaments can be seen after phosphotungstic acid-haemotoxylin staining (Bunting *et al.* 1948). Glycogen is found in the cytoplasm of the myoepithelium (Montagna *et al.* 1951, 1953). The cytoplasm lacks sudanophilic material but is birefringent (Bunting *et al.* 1948).

The Basement Membrane

The basement membrane is more pronounced in apocrine than in eccrine glands. It stains intensely positive with PAS and in profiles lined by columnar or cuboidal cells, exhibits intricate infoldings which appear as slashes (Fig 21) between the myoepithelial cell processes. The infoldings are not seen around profiles lined by squamous cells. Outside the basement membrane is a network of elastic fibres.

The Duct

The duct of the apocrine gland is by general consent, lined by stratified cuboidal epithelium and until 1959, was believed to consist of but two layers. In that year however, Charles reported that the profiles of some ducts could be seen by the electron microscope to possess three layers of cells. This was verified by Hashimoto *et al.* (1966a). Subsequently, Hashimoto (1978) modified his stance to admit that in some ducts the middle layer may be absent. It has been suggested by Montagna & Parakkal both that there are myoepithelial cells around the duct (1974, p 349) and that there are no myoepithelial cells around the duct (1974, p 348). Yamada (1960) describes apocrine glands as exhibiting a unilayered secretory portion, a bilaminar "transitional part" and a trilaminar duct: he did not give his criteria for defining the transitional part.

In my opinion, the duct of apocrine glands is lined almost universally by a bilaminar stratified cuboidal epithelium (Fig 22) but one can in some places see three layers: there seems to be no hard and fast rule governing the level at which three layers are found. Certainly, as the duct approaches the hair follicle, it will acquire progressively additional layers and for a short distance it is usually trilaminar here. I have occasionally seen myoepithelial cells around the duct. The duct is straight where it passes through the epidermis lining the hair follicle, the lumen widening gradually as it does so (infundibular portion of duct).

THE ULTRASTRUCTURE OF APOCRINE GLANDS

A substantial number of investigations has been made into the ultrastructure of the axillary glands (Takahashi 1957; Kurosumi, Kitamura & Iijima 1959; Charles 1959; Yamada 1960; Hibbs 1962; Yasuda, Ellis & Montagna 1962; Munger 1965a, b; Gross 1966; Ellis 1967; Bell 1974; Schaumburg-Lever & Lever 1975) and of the ceruminous glands (Kawabata 1964; Main & Lim 1976; Kurosumi & Kawabata 1976; Kawabata & Kurosumi 1976; Kurosumi 1977; Testa-Riva & Puxeddu 1980). These accounts would appear to confirm the impressions, gained from cytological studies, that apocrine glands from different regions do not appear to vary greatly in structure.

The Secretory Segment

The electron microscope would seem to confirm that only one cell type is to be found here: there are reports, however, that two cell types are to be found in the ceruminous glands (Main & Lim 1976; Testa-Riva & Puxeddu 1980) and in the axillary glands (Hibbs 1962). The now well-documented ability of fixation in cold glutaraldehyde to produce light and dark cells (Dohrmann 1970) perhaps accounts for the appearances seen by Main & Lim and by Testa-Riva & Puxeddu since they used cold glutaraldehyde as a fixative: indeed Testa-Riva & Puxeddu did not see two cell types after fixation at room temperature. Main & Lim, however, did not carry out fixation at room temperature. Hibbs, on the other hand, saw two cell types after fixation in osmium tetroxide, but he is alone in this respect. I shall proceed on the premise, which I am convinced is the correct one, that there is but one cell type in apocrine glands, wherever they occur: the great majority of investigators are in agreement with this stance.

The Axillary Glands

The lining secretory cells have a highly folded basal plasma membrane especially in the intervals between the myoepithelial cells where the lining cells abut on the basement membrane: folds also occur over the area where the lining cells abut on the myoepithelium but here they are less complex. The lining cells also interdigitate where they lie adjacent to the basement membrane (Ellis 1967). The lateral borders of the secretory cells have junctional complexes some 2–5 microns below their luminal end (Ellis 1967). The lateral plasma membrane below the complex is also heavily plicated but here the cell infoldings would seem to be less elaborate than in the basal region: the cell surfaces may exhibit pinocytotic vesicles (Hashimoto 1978). The luminal surface is covered by microvilli. They tend to be more numerous in the hollows between apical caps than on the caps themselves (Ellis 1967). Pinocytotic vesicles exhibiting a wide range of densities lie along the luminal border.

The cytoplasm contains a prominent Golgi apparatus just superficial to the nucleus, and many profiles of smooth endoplasmic reticulum are to be seen throughout the cell. Mitochondria are also to be seen in all parts of the cytoplasm, especially between the folds of the basal plasma membrane where they are usually elongated: elsewhere they are circular and in the apical cytoplasm they can be of very large size with sparse cristae. Profiles of rough endoplasmic reticulum are also found throughout the cytoplasm. Tonofilament bundles may also occur. Membrane-bound vesicles may be seen in the Golgi zone, in the supranuclear region and along the cell surface: these are widely believed to discharge their contents to the lumen by reverse pinocytosis (exocytosis).

On the question of the origin, fate and nature of the secretory granules, there is considerable difference of opinion. There is one school of thought that the secretory granules are modified mitochondria (Kurosumi *et al.* 1959; Kurosumi 1961; Biempica & Montes 1965; Hashimoto,

Gross & Lever 1966b; Ellis 1967; Schaumburg-Lever & Lever 1975; Hashimoto 1978) and another that they are not (Charles 1959; Yamada 1960; Hibbs 1962; Bell 1974). Kurosumi is of the opinion that the secretory granules in *ceruminous* glands are not modified mitochondria, however, (Kurosumi & Kawabata 1976) and this is also the opinion of Main & Lim (1976). It does not seem reasonable to me that mitochondria should here be modified to form secretory granules in view of the well-known function of mitochondria as energy sources: moreover, I fail to be convinced by the pictorial evidence advanced by those who say the mitochondria and granules have intermediate forms.

The majority of investigators would recognise the secretory granules as being of two types (Charles 1959; Kurosumi 1961; Hibbs 1962; Hashimoto, Gross & Lever 1966b; Schaumburg-Lever & Lever 1975) but others describe one type (Biempica & Montes 1965) or even three (Yamada 1960; Bell 1974). All investigators agree however, that the secretory granules are never discharged from the cell but that they break up in the apical cytoplasm and that the contents of the granules are a major composite of the surface band of amorphous cytoplasm, the presence of which is also universally agreed. To my mind there is a great deal in common in the descriptions of the granules: thus they are formed in the Golgi region by general consent (Charles 1959; Yamada 1960; Kurosumi 1961; Hibbs 1962; Biempica & Montes 1965; Munger 1965b; Hashimoto, Gross & Lever 1966b; Bell 1974; Schaumburg-Lever & Lever 1975; Hashimoto 1978). The earliest formations in the vicinity of the Golgi region are referred to variously as vacuoles, vesicles or granules, but there is agreement as to size (circa 0.5 micron), shape (circular), density (dark) and appearance (homogeneous). Progressively thereafter, the 'granules':

1. enlarge until they are enormous (up to 5 microns);
2. become pleomorphic;
3. move from the Golgi region into the supranuclear cytoplasm at large (but never into the luminal border);
4. develop surface blebs; and
5. break up

The extent of the pleomorphism almost defies description. The granules are given the epithet 'rough' because of the surface blebbing by Charles (1959) who describes the surface roughness as spreading inwards. Yamada (1960) describes the granules as having a homogeneous, grey matrix containing very dense and very clear circular areas: he describes the small granules seen in the cell as being derived from the less dense areas of the large granules. Hibbs (1962) saw the pale granules as acquiring a dark centre which spreads out until the entire granule is dark, after which the granules exhibit a many-fold enlargement to become pale again before breaking up. Biempica & Montes (1965) saw the initially-formed granules as increasing in size and electron density before becoming pale and pleomorphic and finally breaking up. Munger (1965b) observed vacuoles in the Golgi zone and at the cell surface: the granules were seen as of irregular electron density both in the Golgi and in the supranuclear cytoplasm, there being a spectrum of density as between the vacuoles of the Golgi and the densest (electron-opaque) cytoplasmic granules. Hashimoto, Gross & Lever (1966a) describe dark granules, of Golgi region origin, as becoming large and acquiring less dense (lipid droplet) globules and as accumulating in the apical cytoplasm: these granules subsequently break up to release their pleomorphic contents into the cytoplasm. Bell (1974) is of the opinion that the forerunner of the large pleomorphic "secretory" granule of the supranuclear cytoplasm is a dark-cored electron-lucent granule formed in the basal cytoplasm and probably in the rough endoplasmic reticulum: a second type of granule, designated as "partially secretory" and found also in the apical cytoplasm is rounded and electron dense and becomes pleomorphic like the large granule but is of smaller size and is found only in some cells.

In keeping with the varied morphological appearance of the large secretory granules described thus universally in the supranuclear cytoplasm, are the descriptions of the contents of the secretory vacuoles at the cell surface in any one cell as being of a wide range of densities. Collectively, the various observations of the granules in apocrine gland cells would appear to be consistent with the following concepts:

1 The granules are formed initially either in the Golgi region or, as is even more probable, in the rough endoplasmic reticulum around the nucleus, from whence they pass to the Golgi region. At this time the granules exhibit considerable electron density.

2 The granules forsake the Golgi region for the apical cytoplasm and are small (0.5 micron) round, homogeneous and electron-dense and would appear to constitute, at this stage, one of the two granule types reported by most investigators.

3 The granules subsequently enlarge up to ten-fold, and become enormously pleomorphic: some parts are totally electron opaque, some are electron lucent (these may be coalesced lipid droplets formed in the smooth endoplasmic reticulum) and the intervening matrix is of intermediate density for the most part: the granule acquires surface blebs which may be composed of electron-lucent or electron-dense fractions. This is the second type of granule described by most investigators.

4 The granules eventually lyse to release their contents into the luminal band of cytoplasm, in which vesicles of a wide range of

densities are to be seen. The granules are at all times and situations membrane-bound and never enter the luminal band of cytoplasm, or the apical cytoplasmic pseudopodia, where present.

The Ceruminous Glands

The descriptions of the ultrastructure of these apocrine glands (Kawabata 1964; Main & Lim 1976; Kurosumi & Kawabata 1976; Kawabata & Kurosumi 1976; Kurosumi 1977; Lucheroni *et al.* 1978; Testa-Riva & Puxeddu 1980) would appear to indicate that they do not differ in any significant respect from the axillary apocrine glands. Thus Kawabata (1964) summarises his findings (in nine human subjects) as being "the same as that of the apocrine sweat gland in the human axillary skin" except that in the ceruminous glands infoldings of the basal plasma membrane and of the lateral border of the secretory cell are "either very poor or quite absent". He describes the secretory process as one in which dark granules, of Golgi origin, enlarge, and become vacuolar (with the vacuoles on occasion forming surface blebs on the granules). He is of the belief that these vacuoles are probably liberated from the granules and empty their contents into the gland lumen. In a later article (Kurosumi & Kawabata 1976) he corroborated his earlier findings. Main & Lim (1976) report that the secretory cells contain secretory vesicles as well as granules of two types, small and pale and large and dark. The small pale granules, they say, arise from the Golgi but they offer no opinion as to the origin of the large dark granules which "are located near the Golgi zone but never in the apical cap". The large dark granules often have pale vacuolar inclusions which may or may not protrude as blebs. The vacuoles, and the contents of the pale granules are liberated from the cell surface by exocytosis, but this is never the case for the large dark granules. Testa-River & Puxeddu (1980) report the secretory cells as "exhibiting vacuoles, dense bodies and complex inclusions": the dense bodies have less dense droplet inclusions and the complex inclusions contain small osmiophilic globules and also lipoid droplets of various size. Dense bodies, or their less dense inclusions or complex inclusions have never been observed being extruded into the lumen. I consider their dense bodies to be the small dark granules of other investigators and their complex inclusions as being equivalent to the large pale granules seen by others.

THE SECRETORY PROCESS

As I see it, the protein component of the secretory product is formed in the rough-surfaced endoplasmic reticulum and appears next in the Golgi apparatus as very small (0.5 micron), osmiophilic, membrane-bound (smooth) particles. These pass to the periphery of the Golgi zone, enlarge and may often assume angular outline, or may be rounded. The density lessens, and the interior becomes pale and is often filamentous. The granules at this stage are of about 1 micron in diameter: they are already showing evidence of pleomorphism. The granules thereafter increase in size up to ten-fold, and become very pleomorphic indeed. Some parts of the granule remain very electron dense, but most of the granule becomes pale and grey in colour: other parts of the granule become completely electron-lucent and may well be lipid in nature and derived from the smooth reticulum. The dark parts, and more especially the pale parts may bulge the granule surface as blebs. The granules finally lyse and their contents pass to the luminal band of cytoplasm in which vesicles of various densities are invariably present but in which neither granules nor mitochondria are ever seen. The granule contents are then liberated to the lumen by the merocrine method (exocytosis: reverse pinocytosis), or by the apocrine method (see below). The homogeneous light granules described by many microscopists are associated with the rough-surfaced endoplasmic reticulum, as are the mitochondria: in the supranuclear cytoplasm these mitochondria are atypically large, round, and lacking in cristae. As such they have been mistaken for granules of secretion – the light granules. Although both iron and pigment are known to be present in the secretion, no correlation between these and the granule contents seem to be possible at this juncture.

Manner of Secretion

Apocrine glands can secrete by the merocrine, the apocrine or the holocrine methods.

The merocrine method By general consent, apocrine glands secrete by the merocrine method (ie. by reverse pinocytosis or exocytosis). Droplets of secretion are extruded both at the apices, and between the bases, of the microvilli which cover the cell surface.

The apocrine method The apocrine glands are so named because some of the lining cells in columnar-cell-lined profiles develop apical pseudopodia: a cross-section through these pseudopodia gives the impression of cytoplasmic masses lying free in the lumen. Some investigators (Schaumburg-Lever & Lever 1975; Main & Lim 1976; Hashimoto 1978; Testa-Riva & Puxeddu 1980) would hold that the cells secrete by the process of decapitation of the entire apex of the cell, and all three incorporate diagrams illustrating the mechanism of the process. Other investigators would deny that this occurs but would concede that apocrine secretion of a less pronounced degree does occur (Kurosumi *et al.* 1959; Charles 1959; Bell 1974; Hashimoto *et al.* 1966b). Yet others would deny the existence of any kind of apocrine secretion whatsoever (Yamada 1960; Hibbs 1962; Kawabata 1964; Munger 1965b). The occasional sighting of the body of a secretory cell being separated from its apex by plasma membranes is explained, by those who deny apocrine secretion, in terms of a tangential section through two adjacent cells: further weight is added to this interpretation by the observation of differing densities of cytoplasm on either side of the plasma membranes. The controversy would, to my mind, appear to have been resolved by recent scanning electron microscope investigations of ceruminous glands by Kurosumi & Kawabata (1976) and by Testa-Riva & Puxeddu (1980) and of axillary glands by Inoue (1979). These show the secretory cells as exhibiting balloon-like surface projections attached to the cell apex by very narrow pedicles. Were these pedicles to rupture, as surely they must, then secretion of a kind which cannot be designated as merocrine will occur. These balloon-like swellings are regarded as being of three sizes: macroapocrine, microapocrine and intermediate. To my mind the microapocrine balloons, being as they are no longer than microvilli, could well be the microvilli with apical vacuoles seen in the transmission electron microscope. There can be no doubt, however, that were the projections designated as macroapocrine, and of intermediate type, to shear off, then apocrine secretion is occurring. Projections of both types are smooth-surfaced. In the case of the macroapocrine projections, only one was ever seen in any given cell (Inoue). The processes of intermediate type are brought about by the fusion of several adjacent microvilli, and the secretory cells will possess two or more, up to a maximum of about six, such processes (Inoue 1979). It would appear that apocrine secretion is with us to stay.

The holocrine method There are two reports (Hashimoto *et al.* 1964b, Schaumberg-Lever & Lever 1975) that apocrine glands have been seen by the transmission electron microscope to secrete by this method. Confirmation from scanning electron microscope studies is provided by Wilborn & Montes (1978) and by Testa-Riva & Puxeddu (1980).

The Myoepithelium

The myoepithelial cells are spindle-shaped and arranged along the length of the tubule (Kawabata & Kurosumi 1976; Mayer & Neurand

1978). They are joined to one another and to the adjacent secretory cells by desmosomes: hemidesmosomes are found where the cells abut on the basement membrane (Kawabata & Kurosumi 1976). The myofilaments are confined to the cytoplasm of the abluminal portion of the cell.

THE DUCT

Three investigations of the ultrastructure of the ducts of apocrine glands have been published. Hashimoto, Gross & Lever (1966a) saw the duct of the human axillary apocrine gland as having two or three layers of cells whereas Ito *et al.* (1976) recognised only two layers in the same situation. Kurosumi (1977) describes only two layers in the duct of the human ceruminous gland: since Hashimoto *et al.* saw the inner and middle layers as having similar ultrastructural appearances, only two descriptions are needed, that of the juxtaluminal layer or layers, and that of the abluminal layer.

The juxtaluminal layer(s) The cells abutting on the lumen have surface microvilli. The cells have abundant, clear supranuclear cytoplasm devoid of the bundles of tonofibrils which characterise the cells elswhere. The cells have pronounced interdigitations and many desmosomes on their lateral borders. The deep surface of the cell is flat and has few desmosomes where it is in contact with the cells of the abluminal layer. (Hashimoto *et al.* do not provide information on the interface between the two cells when this layer is two cells thick.) Mitochondria and free ribosomes are found. A Golgi apparatus was seen by Hashimoto *et al.* but not by Kurosumi: conversely, Kurosumi saw occasional lipid vacuoles, as well as rough endoplasmic reticulum.

The abluminal layer The cytoplasm of these cells contains abundant glycogen but few mitochondria or tonofilaments. The lateral edges show interdigitations, but here they lack desmosomes. There are gap junctions on the lateral borders and hemidesmosomes next to the basement membrane according to Kurosumi, but these features were not mentioned by Hashimoto *et al.* Kurosumi saw the most remarkable feature of the cells of this layer as being the progressive accumulation of cytoplasmic lipid the nearer the cells are to the skin surface. Ito *et al.* (1976) describe Langerhans' cells as being present in this layer in axillary apocrine gland ducts. These dendritic cells possess unique tennis-racket-shaped cytoplasmic granules, and are of bone marrow origin (Katz *et al.* 1979). They are encountered in epidermis, dermis and in the stratified squamous epithelium of the gingiva, oesophagus and cervix uteri, and are also found in afferent lymph, in the paracortex of lymph nodes and at the cortico-medullary junction of the thymus (Drexhage *et al.* 1980). They are rich in immune region-associated antigen, powerful stimulators of mixed leucocyte reactions, necessary for mitogen-induced T-cell responses, and believed to be of prime importance in the induction of contact sensitivity reactions by presenting antigen to lymphocytes (Drexhage *et al.* 1980).

REFERENCES

Alverdes K (1932) Die apocrinen Drüsen im Vestibulum nasi des Menschen. *Z Mikrosk Anat Forsch*, **28**, 609–643

Bell M (1974) The ultrastructure of human axillary apocrine glands after epinephrine injections. *J Invest Dermatol*, **63**, 147–159

Biempica L & Montes L F (1965) Secretory epithelium of the large axillary sweat glands. A cytochemical and electron microscopic study. *Am J Anat*, **117**, 47–72

Bunting H (1948) Cytochemical properties of apocrine sweat glands normally present in the human mammary gland. *Anat Rec*, **101**, 5–12

Bunting H, Wislocki G B & Dempsey E W (1948) The chemical histology of human eccrine and apocrine sweat glands. *Anat Rec*, **100**, 61–74

Charles A (1959) An electron microscope study of the human axillary apocrine gland. *J Anat*, **93**, 236–232

Clee W (1975) *A Study of the Modified or Aprocrine Sweat Glands of Human Skin*. BSc Thesis, University of Wales

Contino A (1907) *Graefes Arch Clin Exp Ophthalmol*, **66**, 505

Dohrmann G (1970) Dark and light cells in the choroid plexus of mammals. *J Ultrastruct Res*, **32**, 268–273

Drexhage H A, Lens J W, Cvetanov J, Kamperdijk E W A, Mullink R & Balfour B M (1980) Veiled cells resembling Langerhans cells. In: *Mononuclear Phagocytes*, ed Van der Furth. The Hague, Netherlands: Martinus Nijhoff

Ellis R A (1967) Eccrine, sebaceous and apocrine glands. In: *Ultrastructure and Function of Normal and Abnormal Skin*, ed A S Zelickson. London: Henry Kimpton

Foster C L (1969) *Hewer's Textbook of Histology for Medical Students*. London: William Heinemann Medical Books

Gross B G (1966) Annulate lamellae in the axillary apocrine glands of adult man. *J Ultrastruct Res*, **14**, 64–73

Hashimoto K (1970) The ultrastructure of the skin of human embryos. VII Formation of the apocrine gland. *Acta Derm Venereol (Stockh)*, **50**, 241–251

Hashimoto K (1978) The apocrine gland. In: *The Physiology and Pathophysiology of the Skin*, ed A Jarrett. New York: Academic Press

Hashimoto K, Gross B G & Lever W F (1965) The ultrastructure of the skin of human embryos. I The intradermal eccrine sweat duct. *J Invest Dermatol*, **45**, 139–151

Hashimoto K. Gross B G & Lever W F (1966a) An electron microscopic study of the adult human apocrine duct. *J Invest Dermatol*, **46**, 6–11

Hashimoto K, Gross B G & Lever W F (1966b) Electron microscope study of apocrine secretion. *J Invest Dermatol*, **46**, 380–391

Hibbs R G (1962) Electron microscopy of human apocrine sweat glands. *J Invest Dermatol*, **38**, 77–75

Higginson J F & McDonald J R (1949) Apocrine tissue, chronic cystic mastitis and sweat gland carcinoma of the breast. *Surg Gynecol Obstet*, **88**, 1–10

Homma H (1926) On apocrine sweat glands in white and negro women. *Bull Johns Hopkins Hosp*, **38**, 365–371

Horn G (1935) Formentwicklung und Gestalt der Schweissdrüsen der Fussole des Menschen. *Z Mikrosk Anat Forsch*, **38**, 318–329

Horner W E (1846) On the odiferous glands of the negro. *Am J Med Sci*, **21**, 13–16

Hurley H J & Shelley W B (1954) The role of the myoepithelium of the human apocrine sweat gland. *J Invest Dermatol*, **22**, 143–155

Hurley H J & Shelley W B (1960) *The Human Apocrine Sweat Gland in Health and Disease*. Springfield, Ill: Charles C Thomas

Inoue T (1979) Scanning electron microscopic study of the human axillary apocrine glands. *J Dermatol*, **6**, 299–308

Ito K, Kawada A, Sato S & Kukita A (1976) Langerhans cells in human apocrine ducts. *Arch Dermatol Res*, **256**, 291–295

Jones R C (1977) *A Study of the Glands of Moll in the Fetus and Adult*. BSc Thesis, University of Wales

Katz S I, Tamaki K & Sachs D H (1979) Epidermal Langerhans cells are derived from cells originating in bone marrow. *Nature*, **282**, 324

Kawabata I (1964) Electron microscopic studies on the human ceruminous gland. *Arch Histol Jpn*, **25**, 165–187

Kawabata, I and Kurosumi K (1976) Transmission and scanning electron microscopy of the human ceruminous apocrine gland II myoepithelial cells. *Arch Histol Jpn*, **39**, 231–235

Kligmann A M & Shehadeh N (1964) Pubic apocrine glands and odor. *Arch Dermatol*, **89**, 461–463

Kurosumi K, Kitamura T & Iijima T (1959) Electron microscope studies on the human axillary apocrine sweat glands. *Arch Histol Jpn*, **16**, 523–565

Kurosumi K (1961) Electron microscopic analysis of the secretion mechanism. *Int Rev Cytol*, **11**, 1–124

Kurosumi K (1977) Fine structure of the human sweat ducts of apocrine and eccrine type. *Arch Histol Jpn*, **40**, 203–244

Kurosumi K & Kawabata I (1976) Transmission and scanning electron microscopy of the human ceruminous apocrine gland. I Secretory glandular cells. *Arch Histol Jpn*, **39**, 207–229

Lucheroni A, Fronticelli F, Spreca A & Gargiulo A M (1978) Relievi ultrastrutturale sulle ghiandolle ceruminose dell orrechio esterno e su alcune giandolle sudiparo ad ampio lume nell uotno. *Bull Soc Ital Sper Biol*, **54**, 684–688

Main T & Lim D (1976) The human external auditory canal secretory system – an ultrastructural study. *Laryngoscope*, **86**, 1164–1176

Manca P V (1934) Ricerche sulla struttara delle ghiandolle apocrina. *Zentralbl haut Geschlechtskr*, **48**, 520

Mayer W & Neurand K (1978) Zur struktur und Histochemie von myoepithelzellen der apocrinen Hautdrüsen der Hauskatze. *Zentralbl Med C Anat Histol Embryol*, **7**, 70–73

Minimatani K (1941) Zytologische und histologische untersuchungen der Schweissdrüsen in menschlicher Achselhaut. *Okajimas Folia Anat Jpn*, **20**, 563–590

Montagna W (1959) Histology and cytochemistry of human skin. XIX The development and fate of the axillary organ. *J Invest Dermatol*, **33**, 151–156

Montagna W (1962) Histological, histochemical and pharmacological properties. In: *Advances in Biology of Skin. Vol 3 Eccrine Sweat Glands and Eccrine Sweating*, eds W F Montagna, R A Ellis & A F Silver. Oxford: Pergamon Press, pp 6–29

Montagna W (1964) Histology and cytochemistry of human skin. XXIV Further observations on the axillary organ. *J Invest Dermatol*, **42**, 119–129

Montagna W, Chase H B & Hamilton J B (1951) The distribution of glycogen and lipids in human skin. *J Invest Dermatol*, **17**, 147–157

Montagna W, Chase H B & Lobitz N C (1953) Histology and cytochemistry of human skin. V Axillary apocrine sweat glands. *Am J Anat*, **92**, 451–464

Montagna W & Ellis R A (1958) L'histologie et la cytologie de la peua humaine. XVI Repatition et concentration des esterases carboxyliques. *Ann Histochim*, **3**, 1–17

Montagna W & Ellis R A (1959) L'istochimica degli anessi cutanei. *Minerva Dermatol*, **34**, 475–494

Montagna W & Formisano V R (1955) Histology and cytochemistry of human skin VII The distribution of succinic dehydrogenase activity. *Anat Rec*, **122**, 65–78

Montagna W & Giacometti L (1969) Histology and cytochemistry of human skin. XXXII The external ear. *Arch Dermatol*, **99**, 757–767

Montagna W, Noback C R & Zak F G (1948) Pigments, lipids and other substances in the glands of the external auditory meatus of man. *Am J Anat*, **83**, 409–430

Montagna W & Parakkal P F (1974) *The Structure and Function of Skin*. New York: Academic Press

Montes L F, Baker B L & Curtis A C (1960) The cytology of the large axilliary sweat glands in man. *J Invest Dermatol*, **35**, 273–291

Munger B L (1965a) The cytology of apocrine sweat glands. I Cat and monkey. *Z Zellforsch*, **67**, 373–389

Munger B L (1965b) The cytology of apocrine sweat glands. II Human. *Z Zellforsch*, **68**, 837–851

Perry E T & Shelley W B (1955) The histology of the human ear canal with special reference to the ceruminous gland. *J Invest Dermatol*, **25**, 439

Pinkus F (1927) Zur Kenntnis der menslichen Schwissdrüsen. *Virchows Arch (Pathol Anat)*, **266**, 422

Pinkus H (1958) Embryology of hair. In: *The Biology of Hair Growth*, eds W Montagna & R A Ellis. New York: Academic Press, pp 1–32

Rolin C (1846) Sudoriparous glands of the axilla. *Am J Med Sci*, **11**, 436

Rushforth J A (1982) *A Study of the Apocrine Glands of the Face and of the Areola in Man*. BSc Thesis, University of Wales

Sasai Y (1969) Histochemical demonstration of alpha glucan phosphorylase activity in the axillary apocrine sweat gland. *Tohoku J Exp Med*, **97**, 11–19

Schaumberg-Lever G & Lever W F (1975) Secretion from human apocrine glands: an electron microscopic study. *J Invest Dermatol*, **64**, 38–41

Sobotta J & Hammersen F (1980) *Histology*. Munich: Urban & Schwarzenberg

Sperling G (1935) Die Form der apolrinen Haardrüsen des menschen. *Z Mikrosk Anat Forsch*, **38**, 241–252

Szodoray L (1948) *Oros hetil Budapest*, **4**, 360. (Cited by Hurley & Shelley, 1960)

Takahashi N (1957) The fine structure of the apocrine sweat gland with special reference to the myoepithelium. *Bull Tokyo Med Dent Univ*, **4**, 259–269

Testa-Riva F & Puxeddu P (1980) Secretory mechamisms of human ceruminous glands: a transmission and scanning electron microscopic study. *Anat Rec*, **196**, 363–372

Vowinkel K H (1931) Ueber das Vorkommen von apokrinen Drüsen. *Dermatol Z*, **60**, 314

Way S C & Memmesheimer A (1938) The sudoriparous glands. II The apocrine glands. *Arch Dermatol*, **38**, 373–382

Weiner J S & Hellman K (1960) The sweat glands. *Biol Rev*, **35**, 141–186

Wilborn W H & Montes L F (1978) Scanning electron microscopy of axillary apocrine sweat glands. *Scan Electron Microsc*, **2**, 245–251

Woollard H H (1930) The cutaneous glands of man. *J Anat*, **64**, 415–421

Yamada H (1960) Electron microscopic observations on the secretory processes of the axillary apocrine glands. *Acta Pathol Jpn*, 10, 173–187

Yasuda K & Montagna W. Histology and cytochemistry of human skin. XX The distribution of monoamine oxidase. *J Histochem Cytochem*, **8**, 356–366

Yasuda K, Ellis R A & Montagna W (1962) The fine structural relationship between mitochondria and light granules in the human apocrine gland cells. *Okajimas Folia Anat Jpn*, **38**, 455–483

Chapter 4

The Applied Anatomy of the Apocrine Glands

The Innervation of Apocrine Glands

There are several reports (Shelley & Hurley 1953; Hurley & Shelley 1960; Montagna 1964; Robertshaw, 1977) that the innervation of human axillary apocrine glands is adrenergic. Perry *et al.* (1955) and Bende (1981) report the human ceruminous glands as being similarly innervated. No adrenergic nerve fibres have ever been demonstrated around apocrine glands, however (Goodall 1970). There is marked stimulation of apocrine secretion by adrenergic agents (Hurley & Shelley 1960; Goodall 1970; Sato 1980; Bende 1981), and an inhibition of secretion by anti-adrenergic agents (Hurley & Shelley; Goodall). There is, however, some evidence that the innervation of human apocrine glands is also cholinergic (Montagna 1964). Cholinesterases have, moreover, been demonstrated around human axillary (Rothman 1954; Aavik 1951; Montagna 1962; Tseraidis & Bavykina 1973; Rechardt *et al.* 1976) areolar (Giacometti & Montagna 1962) tarsal (Montagna & Ford 1969) and pubic (Kligman & Shehadeh 1964) glands. Cholinergic agents also stimulate apocrine secretion (Aoki 1962). In an electron microscope study Uno (1977) showed that unmyelinated nerve terminals around human axillary apocrine glands possessed synaptic vesicles characteristic of both adrenergic and cholinergic terminals. Thus there is a substantial volume of evidence to indicate that the innervation of human apocrine glands is both adrenergic and cholinergic.

Age Changes in Apocrine Glands

The apocrine glands are by general consent small and non-functional at birth in all regions except the eyelid and external acoustic meatus. The glands of Moll, according to Sattler (1877) and the ceruminous glands, according to Hurley & Shelley (1960) are of adult form in the newborn. Hurley & Shelley suggest that the reason why this should be so for the ceruminous glands is that they are under different hormonal control from apocrine glands elsewhere, but they do not give any explanation as to why they think so. The glands in all other situations start to enlarge and to become functional between the ages of four and eight, and this occurs earlier in girls than in boys (Hurley & Shelley 1960; Montagna 1959; Montes *et al.* 1960; Montagna & Parakkal 1974). When apocrine glands are about to secrete, the lining cells are columnar and have PAS-positive granules in their apical cytoplasm in my opinion. Montes *et al.* saw these features in apocrine glands from children of seven or eight: the myoepithelium is also differentiated by that age. Hurley & Shelley (1960) could not induce apocrine sweating by intradermal epinephrine in children between five and eleven however, but this procedure induces apocrine sweating in adults.

There is general agreement that apocrine glands of normal appearance can be found in elderly persons. Thus Hurley & Shelley (1960) have seen apocrine sweat in individuals of 75 years of age. Montagna (1959) saw many normal glands in the axilla of a 78-year-old woman, Winkelmann & Hultin (1958) report normal axillary glands in a 100-year-old woman, and Homma (1926) in the axillae of 75 and 73-year-old men. We (Rushforth 1982) have seen normal areolar apocrine glands in an 84-year-old woman. Montagna (1953, 1959) is of the opinion that ageing causes apocrine glands to undergo cystic dilatation. In my opinion, non-secreting apocrine tubules are distended and lined by a very flattened epithelium, and if the normal-looking apocrine glands one sees in old age are non-secreting, as I think they are, then one need look no further for an explanation of their appearance in the elderly. Winkelmann & Hultin (1958) have described increasing percentages, with ageing, of the presence of a mucin-positive, Best's carmine-positive, PAS-positive diastase-resistant, orthochromatic toluidine blue material in apocrine gland lumina.

The Aprocrine Glands During the Menstrual Cycle and Pregnancy

Several early investigators (Seitz 1906; Kayser 1908; Waelsch 1912; Loeschke 1925) claimed that the apocrine glands enlarge and secrete more actively just before menstruation. Way & Memmesheimer (1938) and Cavazzana (1947) concurred. However, more recent investigators have disagreed as a result of having taken serial biopsies from the same subject (Klaar 1926; Montagna 1956, 1959; Montes *et al.* 1960). Montagna & Parakkal (1974) conclude that "if cyclic changes do occur in the axillary apocrine glands, they are not reflected morphologically".

There is similar divergence of opinion on whether the apocrine glands alter during pregnancy. Thus Talke (1903), Rebaudi (1912), Waelsch

(1912), Krompecher (1919), Herzenberg (1927), Richter (1932), Way & Memmesheimer (1938), Cavazzana (1947) and Montes *et al.* (1960) all conclude that the glands enlarge and exhibit increased activity. Loeschke (1925), Klaar (1926) and Montagna (1956, 1959) report that there are no structural changes which are distinctive of pregnancy. Based on the fact that there is a remission of hidradenitis suppurativa and of Fox-Fordyce disease during pregnancy, Cornbleet (1952) concludes that apocrine glands are less active at this time.

Intersexual and Racial Variations

Schiefferdecker (1922) and Homma (1926) claimed that apocrine glands were better developed and occurred with twice the frequency in women compared with men. Montes *et al.* (1960), moreover, claim that the glands secrete less actively in men compared with women.

Schiefferdecker also claimed that Australian aboriginals have the greatest number of apocrine glands and Caucasians the least, but Woollard (1930) is of the opinion that these groups do not differ. Homma (1926) found negroes to possess three times as many apocrine glands as caucausians, and Aoki (1962) is of the opinion that orientals lie somewhere in between. Hurley & Shelley (1960) claim that the apocrine glands are larger in negroes and produce more and thicker secretion. "Mongolian" idiots lack apocrine glands (Shelley & Butterworth 1955)

The Secretory Product of Apocrine Glands

The apocrine glands produce a viscous secretion which is usually milky but which may be coloured yellow, red or even black, and which may fluoresce (Hurley & Shelley 1960; Montagna & Parakkal 1974). If the secretion be not diluted by eccrine sweat, it dries to a pale plastic solid. The evacuation of the contents of the lumen of the gland onto the skin surface is designated apocrine sweating by Hurley & Shelley to distinguish this from apocrine secretion – ie. the elaboration of the secretory product of the gland by its lining cells, and its liberation into the gland lumen. Apocrine secretion they describe as a "slow more-or-less continuous activity much like the formation of milk in the mammary gland". There would not appear, to me, to be any case for drawing a distinction between the activity of the lining epithelial cells on the one hand and the contractile epithelial cells (ie. the myoepithelium) on the other in the instance of the apocrine glands since it is not conventional to do so in the case of other glands (eg. breast, eccrine sweat, salivary) possessing a myoepithelium. As to the amount of secretion, Hurley & Shelley (1960) state that any given apocrine gland can produce about

0.01 cubic centimetre of secretion over 24–48 hours and that it is then refractory to stimulation for a period of between 24 and 72 hours.

Hurley & Shelley (1960) state that apocrine secretion occurs only in response to emotional stimuli and not in response to heat, whereas eccrine glands respond to both. A very good case has been made by Way & Memmesheimer (1938) and by Higginson & McDonald (1949) for classifying apocrine glands as accessory sexual glands, and Montagna & Parakkal (1974) suggest that the glands in fact produce odorous pheromones. I am in complete agreement with these stances and feel the time has now come when we should cease to refer to apocrine glands as sweat glands.

As to the composition of apocrine secretion, little is known for the reason, according to Montagna & Parakkal (1974), that "the gland secretes only small amounts at long intervals". Hurley & Shelley (1960) demonstrated protein, ammonia, iron and carbohydrate in apocrine sweat using spot tests: they were unable to demonstrate lipids by spot tests. Lipids are readily demonstrable in the lining cells of the tubules using histochemical methods (Bunting *et al.* 1948; Montagna & Parakkal 1974). The iron content of the cells varies widely – "Some cells abound in it and others have little or none, moreover different coils of the same gland may contain different amounts of iron" (Montagna & Parakkal 1974). The iron is paranuclear, supranuclear and, in the latter situation, circum-Golgi in location, and it occurs as fine granules. It is found in the luminal contents only when whole cells are present (Montagna & Parakkal 1974). The literature on the presence of pigment in apocrine gland cells is so confused as to defy analysis, and I shall not attempt to do so.

Some experiments with rabbits are worthy of mention at this juncture. Rabbits have apocrine glands in the submandibular, inguinal and anal regions, and Mykytowycz & Dudzinsky (1966) claim that the glands in males in all three situations are stimulated by androgens and possibly inhibited by oestrogens: they also find the anal and submandibular glands to be concerned mainly with territorial demarcation but the inguinal glands are mainly sexual in function. Wales & Ebling (1972) found that the glands in all three situations in males underwent enlargement at puberty, and that pre-pubertal castration inhibits this enlargement. They found, however, that a degree of depression of gland weight and activity which varied with the region was brought about by the administration of oestradiol to intact males or by oestradiol and testosterone given in combination to castrated males.

In humans, Brooksbank (1970) has shown that four steroids are found on the skin surface of the axilla in men. Labows *et al.* (1979) have shown that cholesterol is the major steroid component of human male axillary sweat, but that the androgen steroids androsterone sulphate and dehydroepiandrosterone sulphate are present in addition, and both can be metabolised by axillary skin to more active androgens such as dihydrotestosterone (Hay & Hodgins 1973). There would, from this evidence, appear to be considerable justification for attributing an accessory sexual function to apocrine sweat: what is as yet uncertain is whether the pheromones are produced by the apocrine *and* by the sebaceous glands, which are known to produce the cholesterol (Worobec & Solomon 1978) and which are androgen target organs (Strauss & Pochi 1963).

There is little information available as to *when* apocrine glands secrete other than that of Fox, Mullan & Thornton (1974) who found a "surge of activity in the morning which is maintained into the afternoon, falling off throughout the evening to reach a minimal level overnight". There is evidence that ACTH secretion by the pituitary occurs in bursts which in humans are most frequent in the early morning and least frequent in the evening (Ganong 1975). There is evidence, further, (Makin 1975) that androsteredione, hydroxyandrosteredione and dehydroepiandrosterone and its sulphate all respond to serum ACTH levels.

As to the colour and consistency of apocrine sweat, it is generally turbid and watery but may be cream-coloured and thick and may even on occasions be green, blue or bluish-black (Hurley & Shelley 1960). It is of not inconsiderable interest that the secretion of the mammary gland may be similarly coloured and that on occasions the coloured secretion emanates only from one or two of the ducts of the gland (Greig 1930).

REFERENCES

Aavik O R (1951) Cholinesterases in human skin. *J Invest Dermatol*, **17**, 225

Aoki T (1962) Stimulation of human axillary apocrine sweat glands by cholinergic agents. *J Invest Dermatol*, **38**, 41

Bende M (1981) Human ceruminous gland innervation. *J Laryngol Otol*, **95**, 11–15

Brooksbank B W L (1970) Labelling of steroids in axillary sweat after administration of 3H-[5]-Pregnenolene and ^{14}C Progesterone to a healthy man. *Experientia*, **26**, 1012–1014

Bunting H, Wislocki G B & Dempsey E W (1948) The chemical histology of human eccrine and apocrine sweat glands, *Anat Rec*, **100**, 51–78

Cavazzana P (1947) Indagini sul compartamento morfofunzionale delle ghiandole glomerulan apocrine della pelle e dell' ascella durante le fasi delciclo menstruale e nella gravidanza. *Riv Ital Ginecol*, **30**, 114–134

Cornbleet T (1952) Pregnancy and apocrine gland disease: hidradenitis suppuritiva, Fox-Fordyce disease. *Arch Dermatol Syphilol*, **65**, 12–19

Evans C L (1957) Sweating in relation to sympathetic innervation. *Br Med Bull*, **13**, 197–201

Fox R H, Mullan B J & Thornton C (1974) A technique for studying apocrine gland function in man. *J Physiol*, **239**, 75–76P

Ganong W F (1975) *Review of Medical Physiology*. Los Altos, Calif: Lange Medical Publications

Giacometti L & Montagna W (1962) The nipple and areola of the female human breast. *Anat Rec*, **144**, 191–194

Goodall McC (1970) Innervation and inhibition of eccrine and apocrine sweating in man. *J Clin Pharmacol*, **10**, 235–246

Greig D M (1930) The analogy of black colostrum to melanhidrosis with some remarks on coloured milk and coloured sweat. *Edinb Med J*, **37**, 524–544

Hay J B & Hodgins M D (1973) Metabolism of androgens in vitro by human facial and axillary skin. *J Endocrinol*, **59**, 475–486

Herzenberg H (1927) Neue Beiträge zuelehre von den apokrinen Schweissdrüsen. *Virchows Arch (Pathol Anat)*, **266**, 422 et seq

Higginson J F & McDonald J R (1949) Apocrine tissue, chronic cystic mastitis and sweat gland carcinoma of the breast. *Surg Gynecol Obstet*, **88**, 1–10

Homma H (1926) On apocrine glands in white and negro women. *Bull Johns Hopkins Hosp*, **38**, 365–371

Hurley H J & Shelley N B (1960) *The Human Apocrine Sweat Gland in Health and Disease*. Springfield, Ill: Charles C Thomas

Kayser F (1908) Achselhöhlenbrüste bei wöchnerinnen. *Arch Gynakol*, **85**, 459

Klaar J (1926) Zur kenntnis des weiblichen Axillarorgans beim Menschen. *Wien Klin Wochenschr*, **39** 127–131

Kligman A M & Shehadeh N (1964) Pubic apocrine glands and odor. *Arch Dermatol*, **89**, 461–463

Krompecher E (1919) Zur kenntnis der Geschwülste und Hypertrophien der Schweissdrüsen. *Arch Dermatol Syphilol*, **126**, 765

Labows J N, Preti G, Hoelzle E, Leyden J & Kligman A (1979) Steroid analysis of human apocrine secretion. *Steroids*, **34**, 249–258

Loeschke H (1925) Uber zyklische Vorgänge in den Drüsen des Aschel höhlenorgans und ihre Abtiangigkeit von Sexualzyklus des Weibes. *Virchows Arch (Pathol Anat)*, **255**, 283

Makin H L J (1975) *Biochemistry of Steroid Hormones*. Oxford: Blackwell Scientific Publications, p 228

Montagna W (1956) Ageing of the apocrine sweat glands in the human female. In: *Ciba Foundation Symposium on Ageing*, eds G E W Wolstenholme & E C P Miller. London: J & A Churchill, vol 2, pp 188–201

Montagna W (1959) Histology and cytochemistry of human skin. XIX The development and fate of the axillary organ. *J Invest Dermatol*, **33**, 151–156

Montagna W (1962) *The Structure and Function of Skin*. New York: Academic Press

Montagna W, Chase H B & Lobitz W C (1953) Histology and cytochemistry of human skin. V Axillary apocrine sweat glands. *Am J Anat*, **92**, 451–470

Montagna W (1964) Further observations on the axillary organ. *J Invest Dermatol*, **42**, 119–130

Montagna W & Ellis R A (1960) Histology and cytochemistry of human skin. XXI The nerves around the axillary apocrine glands. *Am J Phys Anthropol*, **18**, 69–70

Montagna W & Ford D M (1969) Histology and cytochemistry of human skin. XXXIII The eyelid. *Arch Dermatol*, **100**, 328–335

Montagna W & Parakkal P F (1974) *The Structure and Function of Skin*. New York: Academic Press

Montes L F, Baker B L & Curtis A C (1960) The cytology of the large axillary sweat glands in man. *J Invest Dermatol*, **35**, 273–291

Mykytowycz R & Dudzinsky M L (1966) A study of the weight of odoriferous and other glands in relation to social status and degree of sexual activity in the wild rabbit. *CSIRO Wildl Res*, **11**, 31–48

Perry E T, Hurley H J, Gray M G & Shelley W B (1955) The adrenergic innervation of the human ear canal. *J Invest Dermatol*, **25**, 219–221

Rebaudi S (1912) Der Schweissdrüsen – Apparatwährend der normalen und der pathologischen Schwangerschaft. *Beitr Geburts Gynekol*, **17**, 11

Rechardt L, Waris T & Rintala A (1976) Innervation of human axillary sweat glands. Histochemical and electron microscopic study of hyperhidrotic and normal subjects. *Scand J Plast Reconstr Surg*, **10**, 222–227

Richter W (1932) Beiträge sur normalen und pathologischen Anatomie der apokrinen Hautdrüsen des Menschen. *Virchows Arch (Pathol Anat)*, **287**, 277

Robertshaw D (1977) Neuroendocrine control of sweat glands. *J Invest Dermatol*, **69**, 121–129

Rothman S (1954) *Physiology and Biochemistry of the Skin*. Chicago: University of Chicago Press

Rushforth A (1982) *The Areolar Apocrine Glands*. BSc Thesis, University of Wales

Sato K (1980) Pharmacological responsiveness of the myoepithelium of the isolated human axillary apocrine sweat gland. *Br J Dermatol*, **103**, 235–243

Sattler H (1877) Beitrag zür kenntnis der modificirten Schweissdrüsen des Lidrandes. *Arch Mikrosk Anat*, **13**, 783–795

Schiefferdecker P (1922) Die Hautdrüsen des Menschen und des saügetiere. *Zoologica*, **27**, 1–154

Seitz L (1906) Ueber eine mit Schwellung einhergehende Hypersekretion der Schweiss- und Talgdrüsen in der Achselhöhle wahrend des Wochenbettes. *Arch Gynakol*, **80**, 517

Shelley W B & Butterworth T (1955) The absence of apocrine glands and hair in the axilla in Mongolism and idiocy. *J Invest Dermatol*, **25**, 167

Shelley W B & Hurley H J (1953) The physiology of the human axillary apocrine gland. *J Invest Dermatol*, **20**, 285–297

Srauss J S & Pochi P E (1963) The hormonal control of human sebaceous glands. In: *Advances in Biology of Skin*, eds W Montagna, R A Ellis & A F Silver. Oxford & New York: Pergamon Press

Talke L (1903) Verber die grossen Drüsen der Achselhöhlenhaut des Menschen. *Arch Mikrosk Anat*, **61**, 537

Tseraidis G S & Bavykina E A (1973) Cholinergic innervation of the normal human skin. *Vestn Dermatol Venerol*, **6**, 3–18

Uno H (1977) Sympathetic innervation of the sweat glands and piloarrector muscles of macaques and human beings. *J Invest Dermatol*, **69**, 112–120

Waelsch L (1912) Uber Verandungen der Achselschweissdrüsen während der Gravidität. *Arch Dermatol Syphilol Wien*, **114**, 139

Wales N A M & Ebbling F J (1971) The control of the apocrine glands of the rabbit by steroid hormones. *J Endocrinol*, **51**, 763–770
Way S C & Memmesheimer A (1938) The sudoriparous glands. II The apocrine glands. *Arch Dermatol Syphilol*, **38**, 373–382
Winkelmann R K & Hultin J V (1958) Mucinous metaplasia in apocrine glands. *Arch Dermatol Syphilol*, **78**, 309–313
Woollard H (1930) The cutaneous glands of man. *J Anat*, **64**, 415–421
Worobec S M & Soloman L M (1978) Structure and function of the skin. In: *Major Problems in Clinical Paediatrics*, **19**, 7–27

Chapter 5

Apocrine Gland Disease

Infective Conditions

Pinkus & Mehregan (1981) state that "inasmuch as apocrine glands reach their full development only in puberty, they are rarely diseased in childhood". Nevertheless, the infective conditions of the glands may be found then, even if the disease processes are not. The infections of apocrine glands are classified (Pillsbury, Shelley & Kligman 1957) as being:

- apocrinitis
- hiradenitis suppurativa
- Fox-Fordyce disease
- osmidrosis (bromidrosis)
- localised chromhidrosis

Apocrinitis This term was introduced by Pillsbury, Shelley & Kligman (1957) to "denote bacterial infection of isolated single apocrine glands". They describe the condition as resulting from bacterial growth in an occluded gland. Treatment is by hot compresses, and systemic antibiotics if necessary.

Hidradenitis suppurativa is a disease of adults and takes the form of a "chronic cicatrising suppurative disease of skin and subcutaneous tissue first described by Vulpeau in 1839" (Morgan & Hughes 1979). The condition is three times commoner in women than men and is commoner in blacks (Mustafa *et al.* 1980). Whilst the disease is seen most frequently in the axilla, it can affect the areola of the breast (Glass & Vecchione 1978) the eyelid (Sachs & Gordon 1967) the face (Greer 1974), the scrotum (Ray 1977) and the perineum (Ward *et al.* 1974; Morgan & Hughes 1979). It has been shown that host defence mechanisms are not reduced in hidradenitis patients (Dvorak *et al.* 1977) and that the size and density of the apocrine glands are not significantly different compared with normal controls (Morgan & Hughes 1979). The condition undergoes remission during pregnancy (Cornbleet 1952).

The aetiology of hidradenitis suppurativa is unknown (Mustafa *et al.* 1980) and the treatment is unsatisfactory. Medical treatment is largely ineffective, conservative surgery is followed by recurrence and radical surgery is painful and followed by protracted morbidity (Morgan & Hughes 1979).

Fox-Fordyce disease This is "a rare, intensely pruritic, papular eruption which may be considered to be the apocrine analogue of eccrine miliaria" (Pillsbury, Shelley & Kligman 1957). The condition, like hidradenitis, affects regions where apocrine glands occur, but is less extensive in that affliction of axilla, breast and pubo-genital regions only have been reported. The condition is seen mainly in women soon after puberty, but can occur in males. Unlike hidradenitis it can become manifest before puberty (Mevorah, Duboff & Wass 1968). The aetiology is said to be obstruction of the apocrine duct (Shelley & Levy 1956). The treatment is difficult and there is no safe and satisfactory method (Pillsbury, Shelley & Kligman 1957).

Osmidrosis (bromhidrosis) is a condition in which sweat exudes an excessive or offensive odour. Odour of the skin is attributable, according to some, to the secretion of the apocrine, and to a lesser extent, of the sebaceous glands (Rook, Wilkinson & Ebling 1972). Others are of the belief that apocrine secretion when first produced is odourless and sterile, and acquires its odour in a matter of hours after secondary bacterial contamination (Kligman & Shehadeh 1964; Pillsbury, Shelley & Kligman 1957). If, as seems probable, apocrine glands subserve an accessory sexual function and their secretions contain pheromones, it seems unlikely that apocrine sweat is odourless. Further investigation is required into this question.

Localised chromhidrosis This rare condition in which the apocrine glands produce a highly coloured secretion has been "noted and described for over two centuries" (Pillsbury, Shelley & Kligman 1957). The condition occurs at any age and the secretion may be blue, black, brown, yellow, green, red or purple and the appearance of the secretion is often brought about by emotional stimuli. The face, axilla, chest, abdomen and genital regions may be affected (Hurley & Shelley 1960). A detailed account of the condition is given by the last authors. The only treatment known is excision: this is impractical in the instance of a young woman in which the face is affected. The glands must be emptied in such persons "mechanically or by heat just prior to critical social ventures" (Pillsbury, Shelley & Kligman 1957).

Apocrine Gland Tumours

Much controversy exists over the classification and histogenesis of tumours of the sweat glands (Rook 1972). There would appear to be several reasons for this. Firstly, there are those who see the sweat glands of the skin as being of two types, eccrine and apocrine, whilst others restrict the use of the term sweat glands to the eccrine glands. Secondly, the apocrine glands in some locations are seen as modified apocrine glands and are given a separate identity – eg. the ceruminous glands of the external acoustic meatus – and a terminology has been built around that nomenclature. Further, it would appear that the qualifications for a tumour to be described as having originated in the apocrine glands differ from one group of investigators to another. Certainly, if one restricts the apocrine classification to those tumours in which the cells possess apical pseudopodia, one is likely to overlook some apocrine tumours. Furthermore, there are three cell types in eccrine glands (clear, dark and myoepithelial) but only two (lining and myoepithelial) in apocrine glands. Finally, the quantity of pigment present in the lining cells of apocrine glands seems to vary within wide limits between individuals and hence some tumours of apocrine glands may be pigmented whilst others are not. Given these variables, it seems to be necessary to find cell markers for the various cell types involved and it is a step in the right direction that Castro & Winkelmann (1974) have shown that eccrine sweat gland tumours exhibit glycogen phosphorylase activity whilst apocrine tumours do not. It would also help considerably if the term hidrosadenoid could be restricted to the sweat glands proper, ie. the eccrine glands.

Apocrine retention cysts are referred to as hidrocystomas (Monfort 1962; Gross 1965; Holder, Smith & Mocega 1971; Smith & Chernosky 1974; Benisch & Peison 1977) or as cystadenomas (Mehregan 1964; Ahmed & Jones 1969; Hunter & Donald 1970; Hassan, Khan & Kruse 1979; Kruse, Khan & Hassan 1979). In two of these reports (Monfort 1962; Mehregan 1964) there is particular reference to the pigmented variety. The cysts, it would appear, can arise in any apocrine-gland-bearing region. They occur with overwhelming frequency (96%) on the face (which includes the eyelids) according to Smith & Chernosky, but may occur in the prepuce (Ahmed & Jones). The lesion is usually single, but multiples can occur and one case had about 40 (Hassan, Khan & Kruse). The ultra-structural appearances of the lining cells of such cysts leave no room for doubt that they have arisen from apocrine glands (Gross 1965; Hassan, Khan & Kruse 1979; Kruse, Khan & Hassan 1979). One final point that requires to be stressed is that there is a school of thought represented by Mehregan (1964) which holds that apocrine retention cysts are not such but are true adnexal growths.

As to tumours of the apocrine glands, the same terminological confusion exists. The benign tumours of the apocrine glands, according to Mehregan & Rahbari (1978), include:

apocrine naevus
apocrine cystadenoma
syringadenoma papilliferum
hidradenoma papilliferum of the vulva
cylindroma.

They state that some cases of syringadonema papilliferum may show eccrine differentiation. Their classification does not use the term adenoma, which is used by others for non-cystic benign tumours of the apocrine glands. (Pahor & O'Hara 1975; Warkel & Helwig 1978; Weigand & Burgdorf 1980). The benign tumours of the apocrine glands of the external acoustic meatus are referred to commonly as ceruminomas (Habib 1981).

Malignant tumours of apocrine glands have been reported for the axilla (Warkel & Helwig 1978) the vulva (Novak & Stevenson 1945) and the external acoustic meatus (Weth *et al.* 1972; Michel *et al.* 1978; Arato *et al.* 1980). The terminology is here less confused, with adenocarcinoma in widespread use. There is also a school of thought to the effect that Paget's disease of the nipple is due to spread of carcinoma of the underlying breast (a group of modified apocrine glands) and that extra-mammary Paget's disease can result from carcinoma of the underlying apocrine glands (Weiner 1937; Pinkus & Gould 1939) and this has been shown subsequently to be the case in the

1 Vulva (Casper 1948; Dockerty & Pratt 1952; Plachta & Speer 1954; Boehm & Morris 1971; Friedrich *et al.* 1975; Breen *et al.* 1978)
2 Perianal region (Foraker & Miller 1949; Dockerty & Pratt 1952)
3 Scrotum (Parsons & Lohlein 1943; Greeley & Curtin 1954)
4 External acoustic meatus (Fligiel & Kaneko 1975)
5 Axilla (Weiner 1937)
6 Eyelid (Hagedoorn 1937; Whorton & Patterson 1955)
7 Groin (Parsons & Lohlein 1943)
8 Penis (Weiner 1937)
9 Trunk (Weiner 1937)

The association of Paget's disease with underlying carcinoma can occur also in carcinoma of the mucous membranes bordering on skin (Pinkus & Gould 1939) and in the bladder and urethra from carcinoma of the prostate (Ortega, Whitmore & Murphy 1953). Finally, all cases of Paget's disease in the apocrine-gland-bearing areas may not necessarily be due to underlying apocrine gland carcinoma, since Paget's disease of the vulva can result from carcinoma of the glands of Bartholin (Tchang *et al.* 1973).

REFERENCES

Ahmed A & Jones A W (1969) Apocrine cystadenoma. A report of two cases occurring on the prepuce. *Br J Dermatol*, **81**, 899–901

Arato J, Michel R P & Baxter J D (1980) Ceruminoma. *J Otolaryngol*, **9**, 482–486

Benisch B & Peison B (1977) Apocrine hidrocystoma of the shoulder. *Arch Dermatol*, **113**, 71–72

Boehm F & Morris J M (1971) Paget's disease and apocrine gland carcinoma of the vulva. *Obstet Gynecol*, **38**, 185–192

Breen J L, Smith C I & Gregori C A (1978) Extramammary Paget's disease. *Clin Obstet Gynecol*, **21**, 1107–1115

Casper W A (1948) Paget's disease of the vulva. *Arch Dermatol Syphilol*, **57**, 668–678

Castro C & Winkelman R K (1974) Spiradenoma. Histochemical and electron microscopic study. *Arch Dermatol*, **109**, 40–48

Cornbleet T (1952) Pregnancy and apocrine gland diseases: hiradenitis: Fox-Fordyce disease. *Arch Dermatol*, **65**, 12–19

Dockerty M B & Pratt J H (1952) Extramammary Paget's disease. *Cancer*, **5**, 1161–1169

Dvorak V, Root R K & MacGregor R R (1977) Host-defense mechanisms in hiradenitis suppurativa. *Arch Dermatol*, **113**, 450–453

Fligiel Z & Kaneko M (1975) Extramammary Paget's disease of the external ear canal in association with ceruminous gland carcinoma. *Cancer*, **36**, 1072–1076

Foraker A G & Miller C J (1949) Extramammary Paget's disease of perianal skin. *Cancer*, **2**, 144–152

Friedrich E G, Wilkinson E J, Steingroeber P H & Lewis J D (1975) Paget's disease of the vulva and carcinoma of the breast. *Obstet Gynecol*, **46**, 130–134

Glass L W & Vecchione T R (1978) Hidradenitis suppurativa of the breast areolae. *Plast Reconstr Surg*, **61**, 449–451

Greer K E (1974) Facial involvement with hidradenitis suppurativa. *Arch Dermatol*, **109**, 408

Greely P W & Curtin J W (1954) Extramammary Paget's disease of the skin. *JAMA*, **155**, 1054–1055

Grice K & Verbov J (1977) Sweat glands and their disorders. In: *Recent Advances in Dermatology*, ed A Rook. Edinburgh: Churchill Livingstone

Gross B G (1965) The fine structure of apocrine hidrocystoma. *Arch Dermatol*, **92**, 706–712

Habib M A (1981) Ceruminoma in association with other sweat disorders. *J Laryngol Otol*, **95**, 415–420

Hagedoorn A (1937) Paget's disease of the eyelid associated with carcinoma. *Br J Ophthalmol*, **21**, 234–241

Hassan M O, Khan M A & Kruse T V (1979) Apocrine cystadenoma. An ultrastructural study. *Arch Dermatol*, **115**, 194–200

Holder W R, Smith J D & Mocega E E (1971) Giant apocrine hidrocystoma. *Arch Dermatol*, **104**, 522–523

Hunter G A & Donald D F (1970) Apocrine cystadenoma. *Aust J Dermatol*, **11**, 82–86

Hurley H J & Shelley W B (1960) *The Human Apocrine Gland in Health and Disease*. Springfield, Ill: Charles C Thomas

Kligman A M & Shehadeh N (1964) Pubic apocrine glands and odor. *Arch Dermatol*, **89**, 461–463

Kruse T V, Khan M A & Hassan M O (1979) Multiple apocrine cystadenomas. *Br J Dermatol*, **100**, 675–681

Mehregan A H (1964) Apocrine cystadenoma. *Arch Dermatol*, **90**, 274–279

Mehregan A H & Rahbari H (1978) Benign epithelial tumours of the skin. IV Benign apocrine gland tumours. *Cutis*, **21**, 53–56

Mevorah, B, Duboff G S & Wass R N (1968) Fox-Fordyce disease in prepubescent girls. *Dermatologica*, **136**, 43–56

Michel R G, Woodard B H, Shelburne J D & Bossen E H (1978) Ceruminous gland adenocarcinoma. A light and electron microscopic study. *Cancer*, **41**, 545–553

Monfort J (1962) Les hidrocystomes noirs. *Sem Hôp Paris*, **38**, 328–331

Morgan W P & Hughes L E (1979) The distribution, size and density of the apocrine glands in hidradenitis suppurativa. *Br J Surg*, **66**, 853–856

Mustafa E B, Ali S D & Kurtz L H (1980) Hidradenitis suppurativa: review of the literature and management of the axillary lesion. *J Natl Med Assoc*, 72, 237–243

Novak E & Stevenson R R (1945) Sweat gland tumours of the vulva, benign (hidradenoma) and malignant (adrenocarcinoma). *Am J Obstet Gynecol*, **50**, 641–659

Ortega L G, Whitmore W F & Murphy A I (1953) In situ carcinoma of the prostate with intra-epithelial extension into the urethra and bladder. *Cancer*, **6**, 898–923

Pahor A L & O'Hara M D (1975) Hidradenomata of the external auditory meatus. *J Laryngol Otol*, **89**, 707–720

Parsons L & Lohlein H E (1943) Extramammary Paget's disease. *Arch Pathol*, **36**, 424–427

Pillsbury D M, Shelley W B & Kligman A M (1957) *Dermatology*. Philadelphia & London: W B Saunders Co

Pinkus H & Gould S E (1939) Extramammary Paget's disease and intra-epidermal carcinoma. *Arch Dermatol Syphilol*, **39**, 479–502

Pinkus H & Mahregan A H (1981) *A Guide to Dermatohistopathology*. New York: Appleton-Century-Crofts

Plachta A & Speer F D (1954) Apocrine gland adenocarcinoma and extramammary Paget's disease of the vulva. *Cancer*, **7**, 910–919

Ray B (1977) Hidradenitis suppurativa of the scrotum. *J Urol*, **118**, 686–687

Rook A, Wilkinson D S & Ebling F J G (1972) *Textbook of Dermatology, Vol 2*. Oxford: Blackwell Scientific Publications

Sachs D D & Gordon A T (1967) Hidradenitis suppurativa of glands of Moll. *Arch Ophthalmol*, **77**, 635–636

Shelley W B & Levy E J (1956) Apocrine sweat retention in man. II Fox-Fordyce disease. *Arch Dermatol*, **73**, 38–49

Smith J D & Chernosky M E (1974) Apocrine hidrocystoma (cystadenoma). *Arch Dermatol*, **109**, 700–702

Tchang F, Okagaki T & Richart R M (1973) Adenocarcinoma of Bartholin's glands associated with Paget's disease of the vulvar area. *Cancer*, **31**, 221–225

Ward J N, Washio H & Davis H S (1974) Hidradetitis suppurativa of the scrotum and perineum. *Urology*, **4**, 463–466

Warkel R L & Helwig E B (1978) Apocrine gland adenoma and adenocarcinoma of the axilla. *Arch Dermatol*, **114**, 198–203

Weigand D A & Burgdorf W (1980) Perianal apocrine gland adenoma. *Arch Dermatol*, **116**, 1051–1053

Weiner H A (1937) Paget's disease of the skin and its relation to carcinoma of the apocrine glands. *Am J Cancer*, **31**, 373–403

Werth C V, Pardo V, Millard M & Gerston K (1972) Tumors of ceruminous glands. *Cancer*, **29**, 1169–1178

Whorton C M & Patterson J B (1955) Carcinoma of Moll's glands with extramammary Paget's disease of the eyelid. *Cancer*, **8**, 1009–1015

PART II

The Mammary Gland

Chapter 6

The Development of the Breast

Before Birth

The earliest investigations of the development of the human breast were those of Langer (1850) and Koelliker (1852) followed some time later by those of Rein (1882) Schmidt (1897), Schmitt (1898), Walter (1902), Brouha (1905), Berk (1913), Lustig (1915), von Eggeling (1927), Broman (1927), Neumann & Oing (1929) and Spuler (1930). More recently there have been further studies by Dawson (1934), Tholen (1949), West (1949), Hughes (1950), Graumann (1950), Balinsky (1956), Dabelow (1957), Raynaud (1961), Bässler (1970), Ceriani (1974), Porter (1974) and Anderson (1978). Finally, the ultrastructural appearance of the developing human mammary gland has been described by Tobon & Salazar (1974). The account which follows is a composite of the findings of all the authorities quoted.

The development of the mammary gland in the human embryo can be described as exhibiting two phases:

A The development of the nipple primordium from the surface ectoderm.

B The development of the parenchyma of the gland from the epithelium of the nipple primordium and of the connective tissue framework of the gland from the mesoderm.

The Development of the Nipple Primordium

The earliest structure seen is the mammary *band*, a linear thickening of the ectoderm on the lateral wall of the trunk between the forelimb and hindlimb buds in embryos of between 4.5 mm and 6.0 mm. Here the ectoderm is seen to have become two-layered (Hughes 1950). At stages between 7.0 and 8.0 mm human embryos exhibit a surface elevation, the mammary *crest*, on the *dorso-lateral* wall of the thorax and upper abdomen. In this mammary crest the epithelium is multi-layered, and the crest is surrounded by the two-layered ectoderm of the mammary band.

(Hughes 1950). The mammary crest is the human equivalent of the milk line seen in those animals with elaborate multiple breasts.

By the 9.0–10.0 mm stage, the mesoderm underlying the mammary crest has condensed as a single layer of cells which by the 11 mm stage has become multi-layered. At a deeper level the mesoderm forms a second condensation. Soon the mesoderm deep to the mammary crest has acquired three condensations (Hughes 1950), of which the superficial pair are closely applied to the deep surface of the primordium and the third lies some distance below the primordium and separated from it by a layer of loose mesoderm.

Between the 12.0 and 14.0 mm stages the mammary crest (i) rapidly becomes shortened and (ii) migrates dorso-ventrally, so that by the later of these stages the mammary crest is found only as an elevated nipple primordium on the ventral wall of the thorax. Persistence of any part of the mammary crest will give rise to accessory nipples and these in turn may or may not give rise to accessory mammary glands. Around the 16 mm stage the mammary band around the nipple primordium disappears and the primordium of the nipple sinks into the underlying mesenchyme until it (the nipple) lies below the level of the surface. The nipple primordium, initially globular, becomes flask-shaped by the 25 mm stage. At later stages of development between 55 and 60 mm, the nipple area again becomes raised, this time as a result of proliferation of mesoderm, but the epithelial primordium is still wholly below the surface level as a "solid well-circumscribed mass of cells arising from a shallow depression at the apex of an elevation" (Hughes 1950). The nipple primordium remains in this form from the end of the second month until the next stage in its development, that of forming the mammary gland, is reached: there is disagreement about when this occurs but it is approximately at the fifth month. Thus it may start at 100 mm (Langer 1850), 135 mm (Lustig (1915), 140 mm (Neumann & Oing 1929), 170 mm (Hughes 1950) or 180 mm (Huss 1873). Until it starts the next stage of its development, the nipple primordium continues to differentiate in that its superficial cells become keratinised, and the deeper cells enlarge and become vacuolated. Finally, during the 100–180 mm stages, the deep surface of the primordium becomes irregular. In the skin surrounding the primordium of the nipple during this same period, pilo-sebaceous thickenings develop but the skin immediately adjacent to the nipple primordium (future areola) lacks these structures at this stage.

The Development of the Mammary Gland

The mammary gland develops from two entities:

(a) from the epithelium of the nipple primordium will develop the gland parenchyma; and

(b) from the mesoderm underlying the nipple primordium will develop the connective tissue framework of the gland.

At some time after the 100 mm stage solid outgrowths of epithelial cells appear from the sides and the deep surface of the nipple primordium. These are brought about by an inductive mechanism on the part of the underlying mesoderm: and since the mitotic index in the primordium is less than that in the surrounding epithelium, the buds must be formed by cellular migration (Balinsky 1956). The outgrowths, as they develop, acquire expanded extremities. Two or more outgrowths may arise from the same point of origin. The outgrowths from both the sides and the deep surface pass into the underlying mesoderm, which, it is to be recalled, presents four layers. These will give rise, from superficial to deep, to the:

smooth muscle of the nipple
dense vascular connective tissue of the nipple
loose connective tissue of the stroma of the lobules
interlobular septa and capsule of the gland.

The outgrowths pass through the first two of the above layers and do not carry them down as coverings. They carry the third layer down as a succession of concentric layers of loose connective tissue (stroma of the future lobules) into the fourth layer, which forms the dense interlobular connective tissue.

The process of formation of downgrowths from the nipple primordium starts somewhere between the 100 and 180 mm stages. The downgrowths start to branch between the 180 mm and 200 mm stages: again, this process involves cell movement rather than cell division. Similar downgrowths are now seen to arise from the ectoderm of the areola, but these always remain small. At this time, too, the surface epithelium of the nipple desquammates leaving the nipple hollowed out and therefore apparently inverted. By the 220 mm stage most of the downgrowths of the nipple primordium have become canalised by virtue of degeneration and lysis of the cells in the core of the outgrowth: as a result, the downgrowths become converted into hollow tubes, and two layers of (cuboidal) cells alone remain to form their walls.

The growth in length of the tubules continues until, by the 300 mm stage, they exhibit expanded extremities separated by septa derived from the fourth layer of the mesoderm. Amorphous debris is to be seen in the lumen of the expanded ends of the tubules, and is derived in all probability from degenerated epithelial cells.

In the full-term (330 mm) fetus, canalisation of the tubules is fairly complete. They are lined by stratified squamous epithelium where they lie in the nipple primordium and by stratified cuboidal epithelium elsewhere. The nipple constitutes a wide saucer-shaped depression as a result of further desquammation from its surface. Small sebaceous glands can now be seen in relation to the lactiferous ducts within the nipple, and large sebaceous and also apocrine glands lie around the nipple, in the areola. Hair follicles and eccrine sweat glands are found only beyond the areola. At term the mammary gland appears as lobules composed of groups of dilated terminal tubules lined by a simple cuboidal or columnar epithelium with myoepithelial cells between their bases, surrounded by loose connective tissue. The lobules are surrounded by dense connective tissue. The entire gland is surrounded by a thin capsule of dense connective tissue. The terminal tubules at birth in both sexes contain a secretion (witches' milk) and the degree of development is similar in both sexes because this is determined by placental, not fetal, hormone levels.

In the only published study of the ultrastructure of the developing human mammary gland, Tobon & Salazar (1974) have shown that only in the second trimester (170 mm +) can the epithelium of the tubules be subdivided into lining cells and myoepithelial cells because myofilaments are only then recognisable in the latter. The lining cells present in two forms, tall juxtaluminal cells showing considerable differentiation and small abluminal cells, intermingled with the myoepithelial cells and showing a lesser degree of development. In the final three months the gland in both sexes exhibits "remarkable ulstrastructural changes, reaching their peak at term" (Tobon & Salazar). These changes can be summarised as:

1. acquisition by the lining cells of surface microvilli and large cytoplasmic protrusions, and fat droplets throughout the cytoplasm;
2. the presence of homogeneous dense dark membrane-bound granules in the Golgi region; and
3. the presence of finely granular material of low electron density in rounded, membrane-bound cytoplasmic sacs: these, and the fat droplets, were frequently seen being discharged into the lumen.

Tobon & Salazar conclude that "by the end of gestation the fetal mammary glands are endowed with their full secretory potential".

From Birth to Puberty

At birth, the mammary gland is similar in both sexes, and actively secreting. After birth, the dilated tubule terminals involute in both sexes and the gland usually reverts to being compound tubular and lined throughout by stratified cuboidal epithelium. In other words the mammary gland is larger and more differentiated in both sexes at birth than it is in infancy and childhood. Such growth as takes place in the mammary gland in adolescence is only that which is required to keep pace with body growth in general (Dawson 1934).

At Puberty

At puberty, the male mammary gland does not exhibit growth or differentiation to any degree, but the reverse is true for the gland in the female (Dawson 1934; Ingleby & Gershon-Cohen 1960; Bässler 1970). Since puberty may begin in girls as early as seven or eight years of age, the changes may start then, but there is very wide variation. The changes in the female breast, as opposed to the mammary gland, are documented by Tanner (1960) who describes five phases which result in large measure from changes in the quantity and quality of the stroma of the breast. The epithelial changes (Dawson 1934) are also subject to enormous individual variation, and some mammary glands retain their infantile form into the post-pubertal period.

The parenchymal changes in the mammary gland in the female take the form of epithelial buds sprouting from the sides of the tubules of the gland: they arise along a considerable length of the tubule (Dawson 1934). As before, the buds arise not by mitosis but by cell movement. The buds are initially solid but become canalised by virtue of the degeneration of the centrally-lying cells in exactly the same way as had, earlier, the hollow tubules from which the buds are arising. In this way the lobules of the breast really become apparent for the first time. The sprouts remain tubular, although they may have club-shaped terminations. Alveoli rarely, if ever, form at the end of the tubules. Nevertheless, the distended terminations of the tubules have the *appearance* of alveoli when seen cut in cross-section, ie. the cross-sectional diameter of the lumen exceeds the height of the lining epithelium. The new tubules are lined by a double layer of cuboidal cells just as are the tubules from which they have arisen: in the distended terminals of the tubules, the basal layer may no longer be continuous, but present as a discontinuous layer. The degree of distension of the tubules varies considerably from lobule to lobule and the size of the lobules varies within wide limits within the same mammary gland. The major factor behind the increase in size of the female mammary gland at puberty is, however, the increase of the connective tissue stroma of the breast, and in particular of the interlobular connective tissue. The age at which the breast (as opposed to the mammary gland) attains its adult size also varies between individuals.

In Pregnancy and Lactation

The mammary gland becomes fully grown and differentiated only during this period. The pattern of development of the breast parenchyma in the first half of a pregnancy is not significantly different from that of puberty: the mammary gland tubules again elaborate buds or sprouts which, when they become canalised, are still tubular in outline (Dawson 1935). As a result, the complexity of the compound tubular gland becomes enormously increased as does the size of its lobules. The newly-budded tubules are again seen to be lined by a double layer of cuboidal cells.

In the latter half of pregnancy and in lactation, however, the mammary gland exhibits a hyperplasia, a hypertrophy and a differentiation seen at no other time: the compound tubular gland become converted to compound tubulo-alveolar form. The manner in which it does so is again by the formation of sprouts or buds from the sides of the terminal tubules of the gland. The sprouts, with their double layer of cuboidal cells, become distended to form true alveoli of which the inner layer of cuboidal cells forms the lining epithelium, and the outer layer becomes the myoepithelium. The stretching is such that the myoepithelial layer becomes discontinuous. The process of alveolar formation is seen to vary within wide limits from lobule to lobule: indeed, some lobules may never form alveoli, but remain compound tubular. The enormous increase in the size of the lobules causes the breast to enlarge, but there is a relative diminution in the amount of connective tissue, both intralobular and interlobular. A description of the histological structure of the breast in all its stages, including that of lactation, will be given in the next chapter.

REFERENCES

Anderson R R (1978) Embryonic and fetal development of the mammary apparatus. In: *Lactation*, ed B L Larson. New York: Academic Press

Balinsky B I (1956) On the developmental processes in mammary glands and other epidermal structures. *Trans R Soc Edinb B*, **62**, 1–31

Bässler R (1970) The morphology of hormone-induced structural changes in the female breast. *Curr Top Pathol*, **53**, 1–89

Berk F (1913) *Beitrag zur Kenntnis der ersten Anlage der menschlichen Brustdrüse*. Med Inaug diss, Grafswald

Broman L (1927) *Die Entwicklung des Menschen ver der Geburt*. München. J F Bergmann

Brouha H (1905) Recherches sur les diverses phases du developpment et de l'activité de la mamelle. *Arch Biol(Liège)*, **21**, 459–605

Ceriani R L (1974) Hormones and other factors controlling growth in the mammary gland. A review. *J Invest Dermatol*, **63**, 93–108

Dabelow A (1957) Die Milchdrüse. In: *Handbuch der Mikroskopischen Anatomie des Menschen.* Band 3(1) 277ff. Berlin: Springer-Verlag

Dawson E K (1934) A histological study of the normal mamma in relation to tumour growth. I Early development to maturity. *Edinb Med J*, **41**, 653–682

Dawson E K (1935) A histological study of the normal mamma in relation to tumour growth. II The mature gland in pregnancy and lactation. *Edinb Med J*, **42**, 569–598

Eggeling H von (1927) Die Milchdrüse. In: *Handbuch der Mikroskopischen Anatomie des Menschen.* Von Möllendorf Band I. Berlin: Springer-Verlag

Graumann W (1950) Entwicklung des Milchstreifens. *A Anat Entwickl-Gesch*, **114**, 500–510

Hughes E S R (1950) The development of the mammary glnd. *Ann R Coll Surg Engl*, **6**, 99–119

Huss M (1873) Entwicklung der menschen Milchdrüse. *Jena Z Naturw*, **7**, 176

Ingleby H & Gershon-Cohen J (1960) *Comparative Anatomy, Pathology and Roentgenology of the Breast.* Philadelphia: University of Philadelphia Press

Kölliker A von (1852) *Mikroskopische Anatomie oder Gewebelehse des Menschen.* Band 2. Leipzig: Engelmann

Langer C (1850) Milchdrüse. *Denkschr Acad Wiss Wien*

Lustig H (1915) Zur Entwicklungsgeschichte der menslichen Brustdrüse. *Arch Nukr Anat*, **87**, 38–59

Neuman H O & Oing M (1929) Polymastie und Polythelie. Eine klinische Studie mit einem entwicklungsgeschichtlich-historien Beitrag. *Arch Gynakol*, **13**, 494–542

Porter J C (1974) Hormonal regulation of breast development and activity. *J Invest Dermatol*, **63**, 85–92

Reynaud A (1961) Morphogenesis of the mammary gland. In: *Milk: The Mammary Gland and its Secretion, Vol 1*, eds S K Kon & A T Cowie. New York: Academic Press

Rein G (1882) Untersuchungen über die embryonale Entwicklungsgeschicte der Milchdrüse. *Arch Mikrosk Anat*, **20**, 431–501; **21**, 678–694

Salazar H, Tobon H & Josimovich J B (1975) Developmental, gestational and post-gestational modifications of the human breast. *Clin Obstet Gynecol*, **18**, 113–137

Schmidt H (1897) Uber Normale Hyperthelie menslicher Embryonen und über die erste Anlage der menschlichen Milchdrüsen Uberhaupt. *Schwalbes Morphol Arb*, **7**, 157–199

Schmitt H (1898) Uber die Entwicklung der Milchdrüse und die Hyperthelie menschlicher Embryonen. *Schwalbes Morphol Arb*, **8**, 236–303

Spuler A (1930) Abriss der Entwicklungsgeschichte der Milchdrüse. In: *Handbuch der Gynakologie*, hrsg von Stoekel, Bd 1. Berlin: Bergmann, pp 490–510

Tanner J M (1960) The development of the female reproductive system during adolescence. *Clin Obstet Gynecol*, **3**, 135–145

Tholen H (1949) Das Embryonale und postnatale Verhalten der mannlichen Brustsrüse beim Menschen. I. *Acta Anat (Basel)*, **8**, 201–235

Tobon H & Salazar H (1974) Ultrastructure of the human mammary gland. I Development of the fetal gland throughout gestation. *J Clin Endocrinol*, **39**, 443–456

Walter H E (1902) On transitory epithelial structures associated with the mammary apparatus in man. *Anat Anz*, **22**, 97–111

West C M (1949) The female breast and its development. *Ann R Coll Surg Engl*, **4**, 317–325

Chapter 7

The Anatomy of the Breast

GROSS FORM OF THE MAMMARY GLAND

The Nipple

The mammary gland is a composite of a number of compound tubular* glands opening to the surface at the nipple. There is no agreement as to how many such glands exist, and this seems to stem from disagreement about what constitutes a lobe of the breast. The majority of anatomy text books describe fifteen to twenty-five lobes and a similar number of openings on the nipple. Sartorius *et al.* (1977) say, however, that there are only between five and seven openings on the nipple surface that lead from the breast parenchyma, and that these orifices are slit-like and contain no pain receptors: there are other orifices (of unspecified number) which are round, contain pain receptors, and which are the openings of sebaceous glands. Koenicke (1934) described the pattern of openings on the nipple of a breast 24 hours post-partum as being seven orifices at the periphery of the nipple leading from the breast parenchyma, and seven orifices in the nipple centre, the ducts of which "developed branches by means of finger-like processes of the ducts to the third and fourth order without terminating in lobules". From their radiographic studies, Ingleby & Gershon-Cohen (1960) agree with Koenicke about the anatomy of the nipple. Perkins & Miller (1926) studied the nipple in forty breasts from both sexes and concluded that sebaceous glands are always present, that they open to the surface (and never into the lactiferous ducts) through short ducts lined by stratified squamous epithelium: the sebaceous glands normally have between six and eight lobules but hypertrophy in pregnancy to form many more lobules up to a maximum of thirty-eight. Montagna & McPherson (1974) agree that the sebaceous glands open directly onto the nipple surface, but saw some of them open inside the lactiferous ducts. I agree that they can

* In lactation, the glands are compound tubulo-alveolar.

do either. Azzopardi (1979) saw apocrine glands in the nipple stroma and Montagna (1970) describes occasional apocrine glands as opening on the surface of the nipple, and these may be the compound tubular structures seen by Koenicke.

Regardless of how many lactiferous ducts leave the nipple surface, there is general agreement that each duct is of about 1 mm diameter and is, within the nipple substance, dilated to form an oval lactiferous sinus about 1.5 cm long and 0.5 cm broad at its widest part. The lactiferous duct then narrows to about 1 mm in diameter before it penetrates the thick band of smooth muscle which forms the base of the nipple.

The Stroma

Radiating from the nipple to the fascia covering pectoralis major are strands of dense connective tissue known as the ligaments of Cooper. Between these ligaments lies the gland parenchyma, embedded in a less dense connective tissue which becomes progressively more fatty and less dense the further it is from the nipple (Koenicke).

The form of the breast varies widely (Sandison 1962): "The breast of the young woman is an irregular cone of fibrous tissue investing the epithelial-lined duct tree and covered by a fatty envelope". Sandison, in his study of 800 female and 500 male breasts, classified the female breast as being of three main types; atrophic, fatty and normal virginal. The atrophic breast lacks the fatty envelope and is small and fibrous, and often has a lax skin covering. In the fatty breast the fibrous cone has been largely replaced by fatty tissue. The normal virginal breast usually becomes either atrophic or fatty with ageing.

The Parenchyma

The earlier statement that there is complete disharmony about what constitutes a lobe of the breast must now be repeated. Indeed, there is not even agreement about the terminology of the successive parts of the mammary gland tree. Usually, the mammary gland is described as having between 15 and 25 lobes, each lobe being subdivided into lobules. Koenicke (1934) describes the lobes as pyramidal but difficult to separate completely from one another: nevertheless, "thirty-six apices are readily counted". Engel (1941) studied twenty-six lactating breasts and was of the opinion that "it is impossible to form conclusions as to the anatomical form of the lactating breast from . . . the average of a smaller or greater number of specimens". He saw the mammary gland as exhibiting a continuous flow of transitional forms between the extremes of abundant parenchyma to practically no parenchyma at all. It would seem that it is impossible, therefore, to draw any conclusion about what is the extent, the size or the composition of the lobe of the breast in the human female.

The Areola

In the light of the foregoing, it may come as no surprise that the anatomy of the areola of the human breast is also controversial. The tubercles of Montgomery, first described in 1837 when the histological structure of the apocrine glands was largely unknown, are nowadays described variously as being caused by sebaceous glands, by apocrine glands, by sweat glands, by accessory mammary glands and by tortuous lactiferous sinuses. One of the points that seems to have been overlooked completely is that whilst in some individuals the tubercles lie at the periphery of the areola, in others they are outside it. The tubercles are large goose-pimples and produced by sebaceous glands of large size surrounding, more often than not, the orifice of an apocrine gland (Dabelow 1957). These could be described as apo-sebaceous units. Hair follicles in the areola are not usually part of the unit, although it is possible that since hairs characterise the skin beyond the areola, periareolar tubercles of Montgomery are fully-fledged apo-pilo-sebaceous units. We cannot agree with Montagna & Yun (1972) when they say that apocrine glands do not occur in the areola, and Sandison (1962) has in fact seen such glands in over 50% of the males in his study. Nor can we agree with Giacometti & Montagna (1962) that the tubercles of Montgomery are accessory mammary glands. Dabelow (1957) and Woollard (1930) are in agreement that apocrine glands characterise the peripheral areola. We also have seen (Fig 26) apocrine gland and breast profiles lying adjacent to one another in a subareolar situation. Bunting (1948) describes the areolar apocrine glands as exhibiting papilliform projections but he did not state the ages of the six persons in his study, nor the reasons for mastectomy, so the significance of this finding remains obscure. We have not seen such projections in apocrine glands from the areola. Dabelow concludes from his investigations that it seems doubtful if apocrine glands ever occur in the depth of the mammary gland. The skin of the nipple and areola is highly pigmented and in the subareolar connective tissue smoth muscle is arranged concentrically and radially: presumably this smooth muscle is responsible, by its contraction, for the appearance of the tubercles of Montgomery.

THE HISTOLOGICAL STRUCTURE OF THE MAMMARY GLAND

The Pre-pubertal Female

The account which follows is based on the descriptions by McFarland (1922), Fraser (1929), Lee *et al.* (1933), Dawson (1934), Richardson (1947), Dempsey *et al.* (1947), Ingleby & Gershon-Cohen (1960), Toker (1961), Wellings *et al.* (1975) and Pitelka (1977). The terminology used is that of Wellings *et al.*

The mammary gland at this stage is of compound tubular form, and does not seem to differ in its gross form nor in its histological structure from apocrine glands elswhere at this same time. The tubules are lined by a double layer of cuboidal cells and possess a very narrow lumen. The lining epithelium may occasionally be stratified columnar, ie. exhibiting an inner layer of low columnar cells resting on a cuboidal basal layer, and especially may this be true for the more superficial parts of the tubules (McFarland 1922). The lining epithelium of the superficial half of the lactiferous sinus, and of the lactiferous ducts from the sinus to the nipple surface, is stratified squamous epithelium of mucous membrane type (see Craigmyle 1974), ie. stratified squamous epithelium composed only of the strata germinitivum and spinosum.

No report has been published as yet of the ultrastructure of the gland during this period.

The Post-pubertal Female

The time of onset of pubertal changes varies widely with individuals, and there is also enormous variation in the degree to which individual lobules in the same breast differentiate at puberty. Cyclic changes in the appearance of the breast also make their appearance with the onset of ovulation (Rosenberg 1922; Sebening 1925; Luschinger & Centano 1927; Fraser 1929; Ingleby 1929; Lewis & Geschickter 1934; Geschickter 1945; Engel 1953; Toker 1967; Fanger & Ree 1974; Pitelka 1977). In this context it is interesting that Speert (1941) had difficulty in deciding whether cyclic changes existed when comparing mammary glands from different monkeys but had none when examining gland biopsies taken at different periods of time from the same monkey. All these variables make a generalised description of the histological structure of the mammary gland in the non-pregnant adult female difficult. Ingleby & Gershon-Cohen (1960) are of the opinion that the breasts of 30-year-old women are likely to be more highly differentiated than those of 20-year-olds.

Differentiation at puberty, as in apocrine glands in other situations, will take the form of dilatation of the terminal tubules of the compound tubular gland: these terminal tubules of the mammary gland have been designated terminal ducto-lobular units (Wellings *et al* 1975). Their histological appearance will depend on the degree of this dilatation. Where this is non-existent, the terminal ductolobular unit will continue to exhibit a lining of stratified cuboidal or stratified columnar epithelium surrounding a narrow lumen. Dilatation will be accompanied by a progressive thinning of the basal layer of cells, so that this layer will become increasingly discontinuous, leading to the appearance of a simple epithelial lining, with myoepithelium. Dilatation will also be accompanied by an alteration in the form of the terminal ductolobular unit: the more it dilates, the more will it resemble an alveolus when seen sectioned transversely: this will make even club-shaped terminals so sectioned appear as alveoli lined by a simple cuboidal or even a simple squamous epithelium. When the terminal ductolobular units become frankly alveolar, as, according to most reports, they will do in some lobules (especially those at the periphery according to Ingleby & Gershon-Cohen 1960), the gland will resemble the lactating gland. Those who believe that the mammary gland exhibits cyclical activity would maintain that alveoli will be seen most commonly in the immediately premenstrual phase: and at this time, too, the lining cells will exhibit evidence of secretory activity and especially vacuoles of fat in the apical cytoplasm.

There are those who believe that the basal layer of cells in the terminal ductolobular unit of the adult resting mammary gland contains two cell types, myoepithelial and another, referred to variously as intermediate, indeterminate or clear (Engel 1953; Toker 1967; Ozzello 1971). There are also several reports that the cells of the basal layer become highly vacuolated in the post-ovulatory phase of the menstrual cycle (Dawson 1934; Ingleby & Gerson-Cohen 1960; Toker 1967); Toker describes the basal clear cells as being different from the myoepithelial cells and as exhibiting dilated cisternae of rough-surfaced endoplasmic reticulum housing laminated electron-dense bodies: but he mentions that the cells also contain fine fibrils comparable in size to the myofibrils of myoepithelial cells. Ahmed (1978), on the other hand, describes the vacuolated basal cells as myoepithelial cells possessing accumulations of glycogen in non membrane-bound vacuoles. Finally, Tannenbaum & Weiss (1969) report the presence of clear and dark myoepithelial cells. The question of whether there are two cell types in the basal layer must remain open as far as the human is concerned. Radnor (1972) saw myoepithelial cells and undifferentiated clear cells in the basal layer of the tubule in mice. A slightly different question is that of whether the lining cells differ as between the ducts and the terminal tubule. Slemmer (1974) produced very convincing evidence that in mice they differ, but that islands of ductal cells are found in alveoli and vice-versa.

The number of reports of the fine structure of adult human resting mammary glands is quite considerable (Waugh & van der Hoeven 1962; Toker 1967; Sykes *et al.* 1968; Tannenbaum & Weiss 1969; Carter *et al.* 1969; Ozzello 1970, 1971, 1974; Fanger & Ree 1974; Salazar & Tobon 1974; Fisher 1976; Stirling & Chandler 1976, 1977; Ahmed 1978). The great majority of these authors are of the opinion that the lining epithelium contains only two cell types, lining cells and myoepithelial cells. Clear and dark lining cells are reported by some investigators, especially after cold glutaraldehyde fixation, a technique which has a propensity to produce such an appearance (Dohrmann 1970). The clear and dark lining cells do not differ in any significant respects other than that they have different intensities of staining. In view of the wide variation in lobular differentiation seen by light microscopists, it is not surprising that the descriptions of the electron microscopists also differ. In respect of whether the lining epithelial cells show evidence of secretion there is a complete spectrum of opinion from those who saw no evidence of secretion to those who saw some or even considerable evidence of secretion. As a result, it is difficult to summarise the ultramicroscopic findings as far as the cytoplasmic organelles are concerned, but some features are common to all descriptions:

(i) the luminal surface is covered by microvilli;
(ii) junctional complexes are found near the apical surfaces;
(iii) invaginations of the lateral and basal plasma membrane occur; and
(iv) the nucleus is oval and indented.

As to the cytoplasmic organelles:

(i) mitochondria may be few or moderately numerous;
(ii) the Golgi apparatus is supranuclear in location and may be poorly or moderately well developed;
(iii) free ribosomes may be few or moderately numerous;
(iv) the rough-surfaced endoplasmic reticulum may be poorly or moderately well developed; and
(v) secretory granules, lipid droplets and luminal plasma membrane vacuoles may or may not be present.

The connective tissue of the gland is disposed in a loose intralobular layer (which is avascular according to Ozello (1974) but this seems unlikely) and a dense interlobular layer which becomes increasingly endowed with fat cells after the age of about 18 years.

The Mammary Gland in Pregnancy and Lactation

The comprehensive accounts of the mammary gland by McFarland (1922), Fraser (1929), Dawson (1935) and Ingleby & Gershon-Cohen (1960) form the basis of this section. During the first few months of a pregnancy, the mammary gland exhibits both hyperplasia and hypertrophy. The complexity of the gland increases substantially as a result of budding of new side branches by the terminal ductolobular units. Mitotic activity, although not conspicuous, is now a feature of the epithelial cells in the buds. The budding is patchy, some lobules becoming enormous whilst others remain refractory. The formation of alveoli in the enlarged lobules does not seem to be significantly greater than in the gland prior to pregnancy. This is not true, however, of the second half of pregnancy, when alveolar formation proceeds apace: again, however, there is a wide diversity in lobule behaviour. The alveoli at term are lined by a simple squamous or simple columnar epithelium, with a scattered myoepithelium. The alveolar lumen is packed with fluid, cell debris and whole cells, collectively known as colostrum. The origin of the colostrum cells has been a subject of much controversy. McFarland (1922), Dawson (1935), Ingleby & Gerson-Cohen (1960) were all of the opinion that during alveolar formation there is massive desquammation of the inner of the two layers of the stratified lining of the terminal ductolobular units, and that the lining of the alveoli was generated anew by the basal layer. At first sight, this would seem to be the most obvious explanation of how the stratified cuboidal epithelium of the alveolus could, almost overnight, become a simple cuboidal lining of an alveolus now packed with cells. Recent investigators have backed this concept in that they see the majority cell type in colostrum as being epithelial (Gregoire 1930; Engel 1953; Gaffney *et al.* 1976). There is, however, another explanation as to how the stratified cuboidal epithelium of the terminal tubules becomes the simple cuboidal epithelium of the alveoli, which is that, by the distension, the basal layer becomes so discontinuous as to be barely noticeable, and this would appear to be the more acceptable of the two explanations. The basal layer is composed initially of fusiform longitudinally-arranged presumptive myoepithelial cells which in the formed alveoli are of stellate outline: and there are many investigators who believe that the majority of the colostrum cells are connective tissue cells which have entered the lumen by diapedesis across the lining epithelium (Pittard *et al.* 1977; Ho *et al* 1979; Brooker 1980).

With the additional stimulus of suckling post-partum, the mammary gland completes its differentiation. New alveoli are now formed in abundance and the gland secretes frankly. The lining cells become increasingly basophilic. Fat droplets make their appearance in the lining cells: these droplets, initially small and basally-located, move round the sides of the nucleus into the supranuclear cytoplasm, increasing in size as they do. They may become enormous, and are liberated to the lumen. Other densely-staining secretory granules are also now to be found in the apical cytoplasm and the lumen. Even in the fully lactating breast, however, some lobules do not thus differentiate, but remain rudimentary. With the enormous expansion of the lobules of the gland, the intralobular connective tissue becomes very thinned-out until no more than a film persists around the alveoli: so, too, the interlobular connective tissue becomes displaced to the side and compressed by, the expanding lobules.

The Ultrastructure of the Lactating Mammary Gland

There are but few reports of the ultrastructure of the human breast in lactation (Waugh & van der Hoeven 1962; Tobon & Salazar 1975; Ahmed 1978) but very substantial numbers of studies have been published on the lactating mammary gland in other species such as the dog (Sinowatz *et al.* 1980) the rat (Kurosumi *et al.* 1968; Helminen & Ericsson 1968) and the mouse (Hollman 1959; Wellings *et al.* 1960a, 1960b; Wellings & Deome (1961) Sekhri *et al.* 1967 and Elias *et al.* 1973). This list is not exhaustive. From these accounts, it seems that the ultrastructure does not vary much as between the human and the other species. For a good general account, see Linzell & Peaker (1971).

In any cell producing protein in quantity, the following cytological features are invariably found:

cytoplasmic basophilia when seen by the light microscope, after staining by haematoxylin and eosin; and

cytoplasmic rough-surfaced endoplasmic reticulum when viewed in the electron microscope.

The lining cells of the alveoli of the lactating mammary gland are no exception. Fat is manufactured in the smooth endoplasmic reticulum of a cell, and again the mammary alveolar lining cells conform, although the small quantities of this reticulum belie the large amounts of fat produced. The cytological features of the lining cells can be summarised as:

mitochondria are numerous throughout: they are invested by profiles of rough-surfaced endoplasmic reticulum;

free ribosomes, polyribosomes and rough-surfaced endoplasmic reticulum occur throughout the cytoplasm;

small pockets of smooth endoplasmic reticulum occur particularly at the base of the cell;

secretory granules and non membrane-bound lipid droplets occur;

vacuoles occur in plenty on the luminal surface (for a review, see Saacke & Heald 1974);

apical globular cytoplasmic prolongations containing fat vacuoles are found at the cell surface (these detach to constitute microapocrine secretion – Tobon & Salazar 1975);

many lymphocytes and macrophages and a few polymorphs lie in the epithelium;

the myoepithelial cells are inconspicuous and change little, if at all, in lactation; and

the luminal contents are heterogeneous to a degree, composed as they are of whole cells of various types, epithelial cell fragments and secretory droplets of a wide range of densities.

In non-hypertrophied lobules the lining cells of the terminal ductolobular units retain the characteristics of those of the resting gland. Islands of such cells can be seen even in actively secreting alveoli.

Secretory Granules and Method of Secretion

The lactating human mammary gland secretes unquestionably by merocrine, apocrine and holocrine methods.

Merocrine secretion Non-membrane-bound fat droplets are elaborated in the smooth-surfaced endoplasmic reticulum. Protein is manufactured in fine filamentous form in the rough-surfaced endoplasmic reticulum, whence it is transferred to the Golgi apparatus and transformed into rounded secretory granules. The lipid droplets and secretory granules are liberated at the cell surface by exocytosis. Some of the secretion released by this method is, however, pleomorphic, the droplets being composed of a core of lipid with blebs of protein on the surface.

Apocrine secretion The secretory products of the lining cells of the alveoli of the lactating human mammary gland may be released by exocytosis but surrounded by fragments of cytoplasm (Lunger *et al.* 1964). Further, micro-apocrine surface projections form and pinch off. This has been confirmed, for the human mammary gland (Halter *et al.* 1979) and for rats (Murakami *et al.* 1977) by scanning electron microscopy.

Holocrine secretion Human breast milk contains whole cells. The majority of these are connective tissue cells in the early stages of lactation but in later lactation the predominant cell type is epithelial (Pittard *et al.* 1977; Ho *et al.* 1979; Brooker 1980). Whilst the penetration of an epithelium by connective tissue cells cannot be construed as holocrine secretion, epithelial desquammation most certainly can.

The Post-lactational Mammary Gland

After lactation the mammary gland involutes. The process rarely proceeds uniformly (McFarland 1922; Dawson 1935; Ingleby & Gershon-Cohen 1960). Macrophages have a large part to play in the removal of dead cells and cell fragments. The alveoli formed in pregnancy collapse and are removed *in toto* so that the gland reverts to a non-complex compound tubular form exhibiting ducts and terminal ductolobular units. Some of the latter may be so distended as to resemble alveoli, when cut in cross section, as in the resting prelactational breast. Investigators are divided on whether it is possible to tell if a human female has lactated in the past from histological examination of her mammary gland, but the majority are of the opinion that it is not, except perhaps in the case of a minority of individuals in whom some lobules retain the appearance of being actively secreting long after lactation has ceased.

The involution process affects also the connective tissue of the breast. There is a gradual return to normal of the intralobular connective tissue, and of the presence of fat cells in the interlobular connective tissue. The process of post-lactational involution is a protracted one requiring at least a year, if not two (Dawson 1935).

The Post-menopausal Mammary Gland

After the menopause the fibrous stroma of the mammary gland diminishes in quantity and is replaced by fatty tissue (Fraser 1929; Ingleby & Gershon-Cohen 1960). It also becomes increasingly elastic in nature (Fraser 1929). It becomes progessively more difficult to differentiate the connective tissue into intralobular and interlobular (McFarland 1922).

As to the parenchyma of the gland, there is no doubt that it becomes substantially reduced in amount. The gland is of a relatively non-complex compound tubular form, the ducts and terminal ductolobular units of which are lined by a stratified cuboidal epithelium which becomes progressively hyalinised with age (Ingleby & Gershon-Cohen 1960) so that the cell outlines become blurred. The process affects the basal layer of cells initially, but sooner or later affects the luminal cells. It is often claimed that some women carry normal-looking lobules into old age, and that they are more likely so to do if they have lactated in the past. The breast remains fickle to the end.

The Male Breast

Information on the histological structure and gross anatomy of the human male breast is scanty. The ensuing account is based on the descriptions of Andrews & Kampmeier (1927), Fraser (1929) and Sandison (1962). The only ultrastructural study is that of Bässler & Schäfer (1969).

The most repeated statement in respect of the male breast is that it closely parallels that of the pre-adolescent female, in that it consists of a compound tubular gland lined by stratified cuboidal epithelium. Andrews & Kampmeier say, however, that it is lined by simple columnar epithelium; but since they also describe the gland terminals as being alveoli, and since dilated terminals *are* lined by a simple epithelium with a discontinuous myoepithelium, their findings can be reconciled with those of others. The question of whether the male breast tubules undergo branching and enlargement at puberty finds people divided. It would be strange were the male mammary gland to be the only apocrine gland not to enlarge then. It is of enormous interest that the model of a male gland depicted in Fig 7 of Andrews & Kampmeier shows the gland as having some sixty orifices on the chest wall peripheral to the areola: these orifices of *compound* tubular glands can only be apocrine-sebaceous gland openings. Sandison observed subareolar apocrine glands in 261 of 500 cases: he does not, regrettably, give a figure for the female breast.

The lining cells of the tubules of the male breast were seen by Sandison to exhibit globular apical projections indicative of the fact that the gland is actively secreting. This has been confirmed in the electron microscope by Bässler & Schäfer: the latter authors are of the opinion that the basal layer of cells in the tubules contains myoepithelial cells and other basal cells. Richer *et al.* 1977 are of the opinion that the mammary gland in male *rats* secretes actively.

REFERENCES

Ahmed A (1978) *Ultrastructure of Human Breast Diseases*. Edinburgh: Churchill Livingstone

Andrews E & Kampmeier O F (1927) Swellings of the male breast. *Surg Gynecol Obstet*, **44**, 30–38

Azzopardi J G (1979) Problems in Breast Pathology. London: W B Saunders

Bargmann W & Welsch U (1969) On the ultrastructure of the mammary gland. In: *Lactogenesis*, eds M Reynolds & S J Folley. Philadelphia: University of Pennsylvania Press

Bässler R & Schäfer A (1969) Electronmikroskopische Zytomorphologie der männlichen Brustdrüse. *Z Zellforsch*, **101**, 355–366

Bassler R (1970) The morphology of hormone-induced structural changes in the female breast. *Curr Top Pathol*, **53**, 1–89

Brooker B E (1980) The epithelial cells and cell fragments in human milk. *Cell Tissue Res*, **210**, 321–332

Bunting H (1948) Cytochemical properties of apocrine glands normally present in the human mammary gland. *Anat Rec*, **101**, 5–12

Carter D, Yardley J H & Shelley W M (1969) Lobular carcinoma of the breast. An ultrastructural comparison with certain duct carcinomas and benign lesions. *Johns Hopkins Med J*, **125**, 25–43

Craigmyle M B L (1974) *A Colour Atlas of Histology*. London: Wolfe Medical Publishing

Dabelow A (1957) Die Milchdrüse. In: *Handbuch der mikroskopischen anatomie des menschen. Vol III. Haut und Sinnes-organ*, ed W Bargmann. Berlin: Springer-Verlag

Dawson E K (1934) A histological study of the normal mamma. I Early development to maturity. *Edinb Med J*, **41**, 653–682

Dawson E K (1935) The mature mammary gland in pregnancy and lactation. *Edinb Med J*, **42**, 569–598

Dempsey E W, Bunting H & Wislocki G B (1947) Observations on the chemical cytology of the mammary gland. *Am J Anat*, **81**, 309–334

Dohrmann G J (1970) Dark and light cells in the choroid plexus of mammals. *J Ultrastruct Res*, **32**, 268–273

Elias J J, Pitelka D R & Armstrong R C (1973) Changes in fat cell morphology during lactation in the mouse. *Anat Rec*, **177**, 533–548

Engel S (1941) Anatomy of the lactating breast. *Br J Child Dis*, **38**, 14–21

Engel S (1953) An investigation of the origin of the colostrum cells. *J Anat*, **87**, 362–366

Fanger H & Ree H J (1974) Cyclic changes of human mammary gland epithelium in relation to the menstrual cycle – an ultrastructural study. *Cancer*, **34**, 574–585

Fisher E R (1976) Ultrastructure of the human breast and its disorders. *Am J Clin Pathol*, **66**, 291–375

Fraser J (1929) The breast in health and disease. *Edinb Med J*, **36**, 217–241

Gaffney E V, Polanowski F P, Blackburn S E & Lambiase J P (1976) Origin, concentration and structural features of human mammary gland cells cultured from breast secretions. *Cell Tissue Res*, **172**, 269–279

Geschickter C F (1945) *Diseases of the Breast. Diagnosis, Pathology and Treatment*. Philadelphia: J P Lippincott

Giacometti L & Montagna W (1962) The nipple and areola of the female breast. *Anat Res*, **144**, 191–194

Gregoire C (1930) Nature epitheliale de certains corpuscles de colostrum. *C R Soc Biol Paris*, **104**, 1308–1310

Halter S A, Bradbury E & Mitchell W M (1979) Diseases of the human breast. I Selective isolation and exposure of epithelia and their correlative surface features. *Scann Electron Microsc*, **3**, 139–152

Helminen H J & Ericsson J L E (1968) On the ultrastructure of the lactating mammary gland. *J Ultrastruct Res*, **25**, 193–213

Higginson J F & McDonald J R (1949) Apocrine tissue, chronic cystic mastitis and sweat gland carcinoma of the breast. *Surg Gynecol Obstet*, **88**, 1–10.

Ho F C S, Wong R L C & Lawton J W M (1979) Human colostral and breast milk cells. A light and electron microscope study. *Acta Paediatr Scand*, **68**, 389–395

Hollman K H (1959) L'ultrastructure de la glande mammaire normale de la souris en lactation. *J Ultrastruct Res*, **2**, 423–443

Hollman K H (1969) Quantitative electron microscopy of sub-cellar organisation in mammary gland cells before and after parturition. In:

Lactogenesis, eds M Reynolds & S J Folley. Philadelphia PA: University of Pennsylvania Press

Hollman K H (1974) Cytology and fine structure of the mammary gland. In: *Lactation*, eds B L Larson & V R Smith. New York: Academic Press, Vol I, pp 3–100

Holmquist D G & Papanicolau G N (1956) The exfoliative cytology of the mammary gland during pregnancy and lactation. *Ann N Y Acad Sci*, **63**, 1422–1435

Ingleby H (1929) The development of a carcinoma of the breast. *Arch Pathol*, **8**, 653–669

Ingleby H & Gershon-Cohen J (1960) *Comparative Anatomy, Pathology and Roentgenology of the Breast*. Philadelphia PA: University of Pennsylvania Press

Jung F T & Shafton A L (1938) Mastitis, mazoplasia, mastalgia and gynecomastia in normal adolescent males. *Illinois Med J*, **73**, 115–122

Koeneke I A (1934) An anatomic study of a mammary gland twenty-four hours postpartum. *Am J Obstet Gynecol*, **27**, 584–592

Kurosumi K, Kobayashi I & Baba N (1968) The fine structure of the mammary glands of lactating rats, with special reference to the apocrine secretion. *Exp Cell Res*, **50**, 177–192

Lee B J, Pack G T & Schnargel I (1933) Sweat gland cancer of the breast. *Surg Gynecol Obstet*, **41**, 975–996

Lewis D & Geschickter C F (1934) Ovarian hormones in relation to chronic cystic mastitis. *Am J Surg*, **24**, 280–304

Linzell J L & Peaker M (1971) Mechanism of milk secretion. *Physiol Rev*, **51**, 564–592

Luchsinger Y & Centano J (1927) Uber die zyklischen veränderungen der weiblichen Brustdrüse. *Beit Pathol Anat*, **259**, 126–146

Lunger P D, Lucas J C & Shipkey F H (1964) The ultramorphology of milk fractions from normal and breast cancer patients. *Cancer*, **17**, 549–557

McFarland J (1922) Residual lacation acini in the female breast. *Arch Surg*, **5**, 1–63

Mayer G & Klein M (1961) Histology and cytology of the mammary gland. In: *Milk: the Mammary Gland and its Secretions*, eds S K Kon & A T Cowie. New York: Academic Press

Montagna W (1970) Histology and cytochemistry of human skin. XXXV The nipple and areola. *Br J Dermatol*, **83**, 2–13

Montagna W & Macpherson E E (1974) Some neglected aspects of the anatomy of human breasts. *J Invest Dermatol*, **63**, 10–16

Montagna W & Yun J S (1972) The glands of Montgomery. *Br J Dermatol*, **86**, 126–133

Murakami M, Shimada T, Nishida T & Sakima M (1977) Scanning electron microscope study of the mammary gland of rats during and after lactation. *Arch Histol Jpn*, **40**, 421–429

Ozzello L (1970) Epithelial stromal junction of normal and dysplastic mammary glands. *Cancer*, **25**, 586–600

Ozzello L (1971) Ultrastructure of the human mammary gland. *Pathobiol Annu*, **6**, 1–59

Ozzello L (1974) Electron microscope study of functional and dysfunctional human mammary glands. *J Invest Dermatol*, **63**, 19–26

Papanicolau G N, Bader G M, Holmquist D G & Falk E A (1956) Cytologic evaluation of breast secretions. *Ann N Y Acad Sci*, **63**, 1409–1421

Parks A G (1959) The micro-anatomy of the breast. *Ann R Coll Surg Engl*, **25**, 295–303

Perkins O C & Miller A M (1926) Sebaceous glands in the human nipple. *Am J Obstet Gynecol*, **11**, 789–799

Pitelka D R (1977) In: *Histology*, eds L Weiss & R O Greep. New York: McGraw-Hill

Pittard W B, Polmar S H & Fanaroff A A (1977) The breast milk macrophage. *J Reticuloendothel Soc*, **22**, 597–603

Radnor C J P (1972) Myoepithelial cell differentiation in rat mammary glands. *J Anat*, **111**, 381–398

Richardson K C (1947) Some structural features of the mammary gland. *Br Med Bull*, **5**, 123–129

Richer G, Stoliaroff M, Carriere D, Chastenier G & Gromenil O (1977) Etude de la glande mammaire du rat male. *Arch d'anat Microsc*, **67**, 167–183

Rosenberg A (1922) Ueber menstruell, durch das Corpus luteum bedingte, mamma veranderungen. *Frankfurt Z Pathol*, **27**, 466

Rushforth A (1982) *On the Apocrine Glands of the Face and Areola*. BSc Thesis, University of Wales

Saacke R G & Heald C W (1974) Cytological aspects of milk formation and secretion. In: *Lactation*, eds B L Larson & V R Smith. New York: Academic Press, Vol 2, pp 147–189

Salazar H & Tobon H (1974) Morphological changes in the mammary gland during development, pregnancy and lactation. In: *Lactogenic Hormones, Fetal Nutrition and Lactation*, eds J B Josimovich, M Reynolds & E Cobo. New York: John Wiley & Sons

Salazar H, Tobon H & Josimovich J B (1975) Developmental, gestational and post-gestational modifications of the human breast. *Clin Obstet Gynecol*, **18**, 113–137

Sandison A T (1962) An autopsy study of the adult human breast. *Natl Cancer Inst Monogr* No 8. Bethesda, Maryland

Saphir O (1950) Cytologic examination of breast secretions. *Am J Clin Pathol*, **20**, 1001–1010

Sartorius O W, Morris P L, Benedict D L & Smith H S (1977) Contrast ductography for recognition and localisation of benign and malignant breast lesions: an improved technique. In: *Breast Carcinoma: the Radiologist's Expanded Role*, ed W W Logan. New York: John Wiley & Sons

Sebening W (1925) *Arch Klin Chir*, **134**, 464

Sekhri K K, Pitelka D R & Deome K B (1967) Studies of mouse mammary glands. I Cytomorphology of the normal mammary gland. *J Natl Cancer Inst*, **39**, 459–490

Sinowatz S, Wrobel K, el Etreby M F & Sinowatz F (1980) On the ultrastructure of the canine mammary gland during pregnancy and lactation. *J Anat*, **131**, 321–332

Slemmer G (1974) Interactions of separate types of cells during normal and neoplastic mammary growth. *J Invest Dermatol*, **63**, 27–47

Smith C W & Goldman A S (1968) The cells of human colostrum. I In vitro studies of morphology and functions. *Paediatr Res*, **2**, 103–109

Speert H (1941) Cyclic changes in the mammary gland of the rhesus monkey. *Surg Gynecol Obstet*, **73**, 388–390

Stirling J W & Chandler J A (1976) The fine structure of the normal resting terminal ductolobular unit of the female breast. *Virchows Arch*, **372**, 205–226

Stirling J W & Chandler J A (1977) The fine structure of ducts and subareolar ducts in the resting gland of the female breast. *Virchows Arch*, **373**, 119–132

Skyes J A, Recher L, Jernstrom P H & Whitescarver J (1968) Morphological investigation of human breast cancer. *J Natl Cancer Inst*, **40**, 195–223

Tannenbaum N, Weiss M & Marx A J (1969) Ultrastructure of the human mammary ductule. *Cancer*, **23**, 958–978

Tobon V & Salazar H (1975) Ultrastructure of the human mammary gland. I Postpartum lactogenesis. *J Clin Endocrinol Metabol*, **40**, 834–844

Toker C (1961) Some observations on Paget's disease of the nipple. *Cancer*, **14**, 653–670

Toker C (1967) Observations on the ultrastructure of a mammary ductule. *J Ultrastruct Res*, **21**, 9–25

Waugh D & van de Hoeven E (1962) Fine structure of the human adult female breast. *Lab Invest*, **11**, 199–203

Wellings S R (1969) Ultrastructural basis of lactogenesis. In: *Lactogenesis*, eds M Reynolds & S J Folley. Philadelphia PA: University of Pennsylvania Press

Wellings S R & Deome K B (1961) Milk protein droplet formation in the Golgi apparatus of the mouse mammary epithelial cells. *J Biophysiol Biochem Cytol*, **9**, 479–480

Wellings S R, Deome K B & Pitelka D R (1960) Electron microscopy of milk secretion in the mammary gland of the mouse. I. *J Natl Cancer Inst*, **25**, 393–421

Wellings S R, Grunbaum B W & Deome K B (1960) Electron microscopy of milk secretion in the mammary gland of the mouse. II. *J Natl Cancer Inst*, **25**, 423–437

Wellings S R, Jensen H M & Marcum R G (1975) An atlas of subgross pathology of the human breast. *J Natl Cancer Inst*, **55**, 231–243

Woollard H H (1930) The cutaenous glands of man. *J Anat*, **64**, 415–421

Chapter 8

The Apocrine Glands and the Breast

The Mammary Gland as a Modified Apocrine Gland

As far back as 1894, Benda made the suggestion that the mammary gland is a modified apocrine gland. Certainly, the mammary gland is frequently the site of chronic cystic disease, in the course of which the terminal ductolobular units (see Wellings *et al.* 1957 for explanation) become distended or cystic. The lining epithelium of the dilated ductolobular units frequently exhibits apocrine metaplasia, in addition (Krompecher 1916; Semb 1928; Goldzieher & Kaldor 1930; Lindgren 1936; Taylor & Waltham 1940; Foote & Stewart 1945; Higginson & McDonald 1949; Frantz *et al.* 1951; Wellings *et al.* 1975; Haagensen 1971; Azzopardi 1979). The lining epithelium which has undergone this metaplasia is referred to variously as pale (von Saar 1907) pink (Askanasy 1925) or hidrosadenoid (Delbet 1927). The epithelium is pink because it lacks the basophilia of the normal mammary epithelium. The lining epithelium is apocrine because the lining cells are often columnar with apical pseudopodia, and apical eosinophilic granules (Lendrum 1954).

The hidrosadenoid or "resembling-sweat-gland" epithet applied to the mammary gland would appear to have caused much confusion and unnecessary controversy in as much as some investigators would appear to have interpreted hidrosadenoid as meaning resembling true (eccrine) sweat glands whilst others would seem to have taken the adjective as meaning to resemble apocrine glands. Since there is now a strong body of opinion, which includes myself, in favour of not classifying apocrine glands as sweat glands but as accessory sexual glands, the use of the term hidrosadenoid ("resembling-sweat-gland") tissue with respect to the mammary gland exhibiting apocrine metaplasia should be discouraged and discontinued.

Chronic cystic disease and apocrine metaplasia may affect some or all of the terminal ductolobular units in a lobule of the mammary gland:

more importantly, however, some lobules in a breast may remain completely unchanged in a mammary gland in which other lobules have undergone complete apocrine metaplasia (Taylor & Waltman 1940). Apocrine metaplasia is accompanied by the formation of papillae or papilliform projections. I have never seen such structures in any apocrine gland, nor am I aware of their having been seen in an apocrine gland by any other person. Krompecher (1913); Cheatle & Cutler (1931); Lee, Pack & Scharnagel (1933) and Bunting (1948) are the proponents of the idea that apocrine glands are a normal constituent of the breast, and all describe papilliform projections in these glands. They also describe these apocrine glands as opening into the lactiferous ducts of the breast. It seems to me that there is every probability that these authors all saw breast lobules which had undergone apocrine metaplasia and mistook them for apocrine glands: these metaplastic lobules would, of necessity, open into the lactiferous ducts. The majority opinion is that apocrine glands are not a normal constituent of the breast, but only of its subcutaneous tissues (Cheatle & Cutler 1931) and my limited studies of the breast support this. There is, however, a claim that apocrine glands occur in the nipple stroma (Azzopardi 1979) and the Middendorf-Koenicke bodies (see Ingleby & Gershon-Cohen 1960) which have been seen by the radiologists as finger-like branchings to the third and fourth order of the lactiferous ducts at the base of the nipple could well be apocrine glands. Some further study is required and since apocrine gland profiles are encased in elastic tissue (Boersma & Baker 1948; Montagna & Parakkal 1974) whilst the lobules of the mammary gland are not (Azzopardi 1979), a study of the elastic tissue would be very helpful.

Apocrine metaplasia of the lobule of the breast is characterised by the lining cells of the terminal ductolobular units becoming columnar and exhibiting:

(i) eosinophilia in haematoxylin and eosin-stained preparations;
(ii) apical pseudopodia; and
(iii) supranuclear eosinophilic periodic acid-Schiff-positive granules.

The histological structure of the metaplastic lobule or part thereof is strikingly similar to the tubule of the apocrine gland (Goldzieher & Kaldor 1930; Taylor & Waltham 1940; Lendrum 1954). The histochemical properties of the metaplastic breast lining cells do not seem to differ from those of the lining cells of apocrine glands (Bunting 1948; Gros & Girardie 1971; Ahmed 1978). Finally, the ultrastructural appearances of the lining cells closely parallel those of the lining cells of apocrine glands (Murad & von Haam 1968; Archer & Omar 1969; Pier *et al.* 1970; Gros & Girardie 1971; Ozzello 1970, 1974; Ahmed 1978).

Apocrine metaplasia of the lobules would seem to be established for the mammary gland, but what of the ducts? Dawson (1932) was of the opinion that the ducts did not undergo such metaplasia but the reports of apocrine metaplasia in the lactiferous ducts are so persistent that they have to be taken as having some significance. Certainly, Haagensen (1971) and Azzopardi (1979) believe that the ducts show such metaplasia.

Aberrant Breast Tissue

Incidence This is not an uncommon condition, affecting as it does between one and two per cent of the population: males and females show the condition, with females showing the slightly higher incidence (de Cholnoky 1939). Generally, the condition is unilateral, but it may occasionally be bilateral: the condition may entail only a single extra breast, but on occasion the number of extra breasts may run into double figures (de Cholnoky); there would appear to be some racial variation in incidence since 3.6% of Chinese men are affected (Takeya 1934) but only 1.7–2% of Japanese men (Iwai).

Location The majority but by no means all of aberrant breasts lie in the line from the axilla to the external genitalia – i.e. along the embryonic milk lines (see Chapter 5). Thus, aberrant breast tissue has been recorded in the scalp, ear, cheek, neck, shoulder, upper arm, buttock, dorsum of trunk and thigh (Deaver & McFarland 1918; de Cholnoky 1939). The commonest locations are nevertheless the vulva and the axilla and compendia of the instances of accessory breasts in the former location by Garcia *et al.* (1978) and in the latter by de Cholnoky (1951) can be consulted for further details. In the vulva, both the labia majora and the labia minora are recorded as sites of ectopic breasts.

Classification All degrees of development from the presence of mere nipples (polythelia) through to a fully-developed and fully-functional breast with nipple and areola are recorded. Kajava (1915) subdivides supernumerary breasts in all regions into eight categories whereas de Cholnoky (1951) recognises only four classes of *axillary* supernumerary breasts.

Significance The supernumerary breast is usually of no clinical importance, but some patients may request resection for personal reasons or because of enlargement in pregnancy, which is a common occurrence. The accessory breast may lactate (ie. produce a milky fluid) in pregnancy, and this presupposes that it has a duct leading to the exterior: if it has not, it may form a cyst, especially in pregnancy. Thus de Cholnoky

(1951) in his study of 90 cases of axillary breast, found normal breast tissue in 34.6% and cystic disease in 38.5%. The final significance of accessory breast tissue is that it may be the seat of tumour formation: this occurs only in those supernumerary breasts which possess glandular tissue (de Cholnoky 1939). The tumours recorded are fibroadenoma, cystic fibroadenoma and carcinoma, but all are rare.

The fact that supernumerary breasts are commonest in those regions in which apocrine glands are commonest (axilla, milk lines, external genitalia) and that they occur in widespread skin regions which are far removed from the milk lines but in which apocrine glands are known to occur, may suggest that some case of supernumerary breast may represent metaplasia of apocrine glands to mammary glands. This interpretation receives reinforcement from de Cholnoky's observation that some aberrant breasts consist only of glandular tissue and ducts – ie. there is no nipple or areola. This interpretation would also mean that not all cases of aberrant breasts are congenital, as is generally thought.

Breast Tumours as Evidence of the Breast Being a Modified Apocrine Gland

Dawson (1932) and Lee, Pack & Scharnagel (1933) presented long and well-documented accounts of "sweat gland cancer of the breast". The lesions were characterised by cells which were pale, eosinophilic and possessed apical cytoplasmic projections, and strong arguments were advanced in favour of there being a normal complement of apocrine "sweat" glands in the breast, and which were the seat of the malignant change. Later Higginson & McDonald (1949) claimed that such pale epithelium is a normal constituent of every breast "if diligently sought after" and that it occurs in "any and all female breasts after the age of puberty". They concluded that the function of this pale apocrine epithelium was of an accessory sexual nature "to impart the characteristic mammalian, racial and individual odour or odours to the milk". In the earlier part of this book I have advanced the opinion that such apocrine appearances in the breast are due to apocrine metaplasia after cystic change, and that apocrine glands are not normally present in the breast, and that most modern authorities agree with this stance. Apocrine carcinoma of the breast is recognised as an entity in modern texts on the mammary gland (Bonser *et al.* 1961; Haagensen 1971; Azzopardi 1979) and the ultrastructural appearances of the tumour cells resemble those of the lining cells of apocrine glands (Frable & Kay 1968; Ahmed 1978; Mossler *et al.* 1980; Roddy & Silverberg 1980). Apocrine carcinoma was seen in only six (0.4%) of 1500 cases of breast carcinoma (Mossler *et al.*) but the diagnosis was based on the presence of eosinophilic granular epithelium *and apical pseudopodia* (my italics). Anyone who has read the early part of this book will realise that the lining cells of the majority of apocrine glands do not possess apical pseudopodia, and so it is very probable that the figures from Mossler *et al.* could represent an understatement of the frequency of occurrence of apocrine carcinoma – ie. of carcinoma in a breast lobule that has earlier undergone apocrine metaplasia. All in all, however, the evidence from the pathology of the breast in tumour formation adds further weight of evidence to the case for the mammary gland being a modified apocrine gland.

Coloured Milk

The secretory product of the apocrine glands is normally turbid, but may be white, blue green or bluish-black (Hurley & Shelley 1960). The fluid secreted by the mammary gland is normally white. However, it may be blue, black or yellow, and the coloured milk has been reported as issuing from two lactiferous ducts but not from others (Greig 1930).

REFERENCES

Ahmed A (1978) *Atlas of the Ultrastructure of Breast Diseases*. Edinburgh: Churchill Livingstone

Archer F & Omar M (1969) Pink cell metaplasia in a fibroadenoma of the human breast. *J Pathol Bacteriol*, **99**, 119–124

Askanasy M (1925) *Schweiz Med Wochenschr*, **6**, 1017

Azzopardi J G (1979) *Problems in Breast Pathology* London: W B Saunders Co

Benda C (1894) Das Verhaeltnis der Milchdrüse zu den Hautdrüsen. *Dermatol Z*, **1**, 94

Boersma D & Baker B L (1948) Sites of deposition of silver in argyria. *Arch Dermatol Syphilol*, **57**, 1009–1012

Bonser G M, Dossett J A & Jull J N (1961) *Human and Experimental Breast Cancer*. London: Pitman Medical

Bunting H (1948) Cytochemical properties of apocrine glands normally present in the human mammary gland. *Anat Rec*, **101**, 5–12

Cheatle G L & Cutler M (1931) *Tumours of the Breast*. London: Edward Arnold

Cholnoky T de (1939) Supernumerary breast. *Arch Surg*, **39**, 926–941

Cholnoky T de (1951) Accessory breast tissue in the axilla. *N Y State J Med*, **51**, 2245–2248

Dawson E K (1932) Sweat gland carcinoma of the breast. *Edinb Med J*, **39**, 409–438

Deaver J B & McFarland J (1918) *The Breast. Its Anomalies and Diseases and their Treatment*. London: William Heinemann

Delbet P (1927) *Les Cancers du Sein*. Paris

Ewing J (1940) *Neoplastic Diseases*. Philadelphia PA: W B Saunders Co

Foote F W & Stewart F W (1945) Comparative studies of cancerous vs non-cancerous breasts. *Ann Surg*, **121**, 6–53

Frable W J & Kay S (1968) Carcinoma of the breast. Histologic and clinical features of apocrine tumours. *Cancer*, **21**, 756–763

Frantz V K, Pickren J W, Melcher G W & Auchinloss H (1951) Incidence of chronic cystic disease in so-called normal breasts. *Cancer*, **4**, 762–783

Garcia J C, Verkauf B S, Hochberg C J & Ingram J M (1978) Aberrant breast tissue of the vulva. A case report and review of the literature. *Obstet Gynecol*, **52**, 225–228

Goldzieher M A & Kaldor J (1930) Cystic cirrhosis of the breast. *Arch Surg*, **20**, 473–490

Greig D M (1930) The analogy of black colostrum to melanhidrosis, with some remarks on coloured milk and coloured sweat. *Edinb Med J*, **37**, 524–544

Gros C M & Girardie J (1971) Les glandes apocrines axillaires et la metaplasie hidrosadenoide mammaire. Comparaison histochimique et ultrastructurale. *Ann Histochem*, **16**, 9–27

Haagensen C D (1971) *Diseases of the Breast*. Philadelphia PA: W B Saunders Co

Higginson J F & McDonald J R (1949) Apocrine tissue, chronic cystic mastitis and sweat gland carcinoma of the breast. *Surg Gynecol Obstet*, **88**, 1–10

Ingleby H & Gershon-Cohen J (1960) *Comparative Anatomy, Pathology and Roentgenology of the Breast*. Philadelphia PA: University of Pennsylvania Press

Iwai, cited by de Cholnoky, 1939

Kajava Y (1915) The proportion of supernumerary nipples in the Finnish population. *Duodecim*, **31**, 143

Krompecher E (1916) *Verh Dtsch Pathol Ges*, **16**, 365–384

Lee B J, Pack G T & Scharnagel I (1933) Sweat gland cancer of the breast. *Surg Gynecol Obstet*, **56**, 975–996

Lendrum A C (1954) On the pink epithelium of the cystic breast and staining of its granules. *J Pathol Bacteriol*, **57**, 267–270

Lindgren S (1936) On mastopathica cystica. *Acta Chir Scand*, **79**, 119–140

Montagna W & Parakkal P F (1974) *The Structure and Function of Skin*. New York: Academic Press

Mossler J A, Barton T K, Brinkhous A D, McCarty K S, Moylan J A & McCarty K S Jnr (1980) Apocrine differentiation in human mammary carcinoma. *Cancer*, **46**, 2463–2471

Murad T M & von Haam E (1968) The ultrastructure of fibrocystic disease of the breast. *Cancer*, **22**, 587–600

Ozzello L (1971) Ultrastructure of the human mammary gland. *Pathology Annual*, ed S C Sommers. New York: Appleton-Century-Crofts

Ozzello L (1974) Electron microscope study of functional and dysfunctional human mammary glands. *J Invest Dermatol*, **63**, 19–26

Pier W J, Garancis J C & Kuzma J F (1970) The ultrastructure of apocrine cells in intracystic papilloma and fibrocystic disease of the breast. *Arch Pathol*, **89**, 446–452

Roddy H J & Silverberg S G (1980) Ultrastructural analysis of apocrine carcinoma of the human breast. *Ultrastruct Pathol*, **1**, 385–393

Saar, von (1907) *Arch Clin Chir*, **84**, 223

Semb C (1928) *Acta Chir Scand*, **64**, 1–484

Takeya S (1934) Ueber die überzähligen Brustwarzen bei Chinesen. *J Orient Med*, **20**, 32A

Taylor H C & Waltham C A (1940) Hyperplasias of the mammary gland in the human being and the mouse. *Arch Surg*, **40**, 733–755

Wellings S R, Jensen H M & Marcum R G (1975) An atlas of subgross pathology of the human breast with special reference to precancerous lesions. *J Natl Cancer Inst*, **55**, 231–273

Index